Embedded
First Responder
Chaplaincy

Embedded
First Responder
Chaplaincy

Caring for Our Most Valuable
and Vulnerable Public Servants

Glenn Davis, MDiv
Atrium Health Wake Forest Baptist

Teresa Cutts, PhD
Wake Forest School of Medicine

Stakeholder Press
BOOKS TO MAKE THE WORLD BETTER

Chaplain Glenn Davis

principal contact

chaplaindavis@gmail.com

ISBN: 978-1-7324222-5-4

Stakeholder Press is the publishing arm of Stakeholder Health in Winston-Salem, NC. All profits from the sale of this book support the educational work of Stakeholder Health. For more information about both Stakeholder Health and Stakeholder Press, visit www.stakeholderhealth.org.

Printed in the United States of America

This book is printed on archival-quality paper that meets requirements of the American National Standard for Information Sciences, Permanence of Paper, Printed Library Materials, ANSI Z39.48-1984.

Contents

Preface

A Week in the Life
of the First Responder Chaplaincy Team

On an early summer morning, 2021, the FRC Team's Program Director received a call from an EMS supervisor, requesting chaplaincy support for multiple First Responders who still involved with a pediatric call involving what would later reveal to be the homicidal death of a five year old. This child's death embodied all of the most distressing elements for First Responders, including extremely high levels of sensory exposure that involved not only seeing the fatal injuries up close but also wrestling with their own anger, all the while questioning how any adult could inflict such egregious harm and suffering upon a child. However, many other staff from multiple agencies involved with the welfare of the child were also heavily impacted and left with feelings of their own anger and guilt about how this could happen to an innocent child.

The following day, the FRC Team met with all affected staff, including First Responders of multiple agencies, some of whom had responded to a second juvenile death earlier that day.

In addition to the 20 calls that come the next day to all FRC Team members, the Director is also briefed at a weekly command level staff meeting of numerous crises (crimes, accidents, injuries and deaths) that have occurred throughout the community, many of which also impact the First Responders themselves and their

This child's death embodied all of the most distressing elements for First Responders, including extremely high levels of sensory exposure that involved not only seeing the fatal injuries up close but also wrestling with their own anger, all the while questioning how any adult could inflict such egregious harm and suffering upon a child.

families. These needs are immediately relayed to the FRC Team which responds expeditiously to each referral. This level of hyper-vigilance with respect to both monitoring and addressing needs as soon as they are discovered is a routine day's work for the FRC Team which sees this large extended family as a parish without walls. Several First Responder retirees are grappling with serious illness. One retiree was recently diagnosed with a rare metastatic cancer, sad news that also affected not just loved ones, but many retiree peers who are dealing with their own challenges. The FRC Team regularly posts these various needs within the First Responder family on a PDF document that is disseminated via email to foster support and empathy within the entire agency, but only with permission. (More about this document, the Hospital-Carelist, can be found in the glossary). However, in this case the FRC Team honors the request for confidentiality but immediately begins laying the groundwork for a broader web of support that the retiree and his family will need during the course of extensive treatment.

Late Thursday of the same week, the Program Director received a call from a Public Health (PH) supervisor, who reported that two long-term staff members, while on a routine inspection of a local business, had just been physically threatened and terrified by the owner who also brandished a handgun. Within an hour, a FRC Team member was on site to conduct a group crisis intervention (GCI) with the impacted staff members and their supervisors and develop a plan for follow-up care. (See page 93 for an in-depth case study of this event.)

There were two other deaths that weekend, one related to a high-speed motor vehicle accident, in which the driver was hor-ribly mutilated and another involving a local government employee killed tragically in an on-the-job accident, crushed to death by machinery. These tragic deaths expose both First Responders and bystanders without warning to the most graphic of images caused by body mutilation and contortion, gruesome blunt force injuries and burns, property destruction and more. Viewing and dealing with these scenes can result in some of the most harmful critical incident stress for First Responders, but especially for survivors-victims-witnesses who have no training nor prior experience in coping with these horrific scenes.

Another critical incident the following day had more far-reaching repercussions and led to the activation of the entire FRC Team, a decision the Director calls an "all hands on deck" call. This incident involved a lone assailant, armed with an assault rifle, attacking a law enforcement district office during shift change when more law enforcement officers would be on site. Even though the assailant fired dozens of rounds into the building, no officers were injured in this barrage of gunfire, nor in the protracted incident that lasted hours and culminated in a popular city park, endangering many civilians, and involving over a hundred law enforcement officers.

In the ensuing investigation while searching for a motive, officers discovered that the assailant had shot and killed two close family members at two different locations before the attack on the law enforcement district office.

Disruptions over many hours during that day were immense along with extensive media coverage. The FRC Team provided immediate on-scene support and follow-up care to impacted officers and Telecommunicators who were involved with this difficult incident. (See page 99 for an in-depth case study of this event.)

Readers probably need to stop and check their own pulse after reading about this *just one work week* in the life of the FRC Team. Take a cleansing breath and we'll now move to share more background and history of the FRCP.

Another critical incident the following day had more far-reaching repercussions and led to the activation of the entire FRC Team, a decision the Director calls an "all hands on deck" call.

First Responders serve and protect us daily often putting their health and even their lives in peril. Yet the public that relies constantly on their vigilance and skills understand little of the sacrifices they endure for our benefit.

Introduction

First Responders comprise a large and tightly interwoven family linked with one another across the nation. Collectively, they are our most valuable but also most vulnerable public servants. The many stressors accompanying their unique jobs are life-altering and greatly impact the quality of life for them and their families. First Responders serve and protect us daily often putting their health and even their lives in peril. Yet the public that relies constantly on their vigilance and skills understand little of the sacrifices they endure for our benefit.

First Responders include those actively serving in both paid and volunteer capacities within the professions of law enforcement and emergency services (which includes emergency medical services or EMS and the fire service).

This book shares in depth the work of the Atrium Health Wake Forest Baptist's First Responder Chaplaincy Program's (FRCP) team members, who essentially function as First Responders to the First Responders. It includes the FRCP's history, development, staffing and training, and is a comprehensive, descriptive and quantitative effort to highlight and value its work. However, to give the reader a clearer view of what comprises an actual recent week of work and experiences for the FRC Team, we started with the events described in the Preface. (See Appendix 1 for a glossary of commonly-used terms, including acronyms and definitions.)

Background on First Responder Needs

The FRCP's hospital-based/ community focused and embedded model is where the innovation occurs, along with the multi-partner collaboration.

First Responders, particularly those actively serving, are subject to acute and chronic stressors daily in the performance of their duties that can adversely impact their physical and mental health along with morale, productivity and job retention within their respective agencies. Additionally, there is growing evidence that First Responders are at higher risk of suicide (up to 46.8% lifetime prevalence of suicidal ideation in one study),[1] and often cope with overuse or abuse of alcohol and other substances and suffer unnecessarily from preventable lifestyle-related illnesses, such as heart disease, diabetes and obesity.[2] This work is not intended to provide an academic review of First Responder stress or health status. However, see Appendix 2 for a more comprehensive listing of recent key academic references on these topics.

The FRC Team's services, in caring for the whole person, promote individual and organizational wellness. The team also provides First Responders with the ability to access chaplaincy services directly and confidentially, whether on or off duty, to obtain support and crisis intervention services for them and their families, and, when necessary, access additional referral resources, such as mental health or financial help.

First Responders also regularly use the FRC Team on callouts involving death and other tragedies to deliver traumatic messages and provide a range of other on-scene assistance to survivors-victims-witnesses of crime and other trauma. This additional use of the FRC Team's services is critical as it frees up First Responders to attend to other essential on-scene tasks (investigations, evidence collection, interviewing, etc.), while knowing that professional, competent, compassionate on-scene care is being provided by the FRC Team to family members, and often to neighbors and other witnesses who are dealing with traumatic grief.

The FRCP's hospital-based/community focused and embedded model is where the innovation occurs, along with the multi-partner collaboration. Overwhelmingly, "chaplaincy," outside of hospitals (with the main exceptions existing in state/federal prisons, some corporate settings and the military), is a voluntary enterprise rife with many disparities, that include among others, limited or no funding, insufficient training and deep entanglements with regards to religious indoctrination and/or politicization in the agencies being served.

To help the reader better understand First Responders, it is important to highlight several of the challenges they currently face in their multi-faceted roles. In addition to being inherently dangerous, both physically and emotionally, the work of First Responders can be exceedingly complex, filled with role shifts and experiences, many of which are never fully processed but impact the First Responders and their families.

As just one example of the complexity for law enforcement, every criminal incident automatically involves the CJS (criminal justice system). The incident itself and the ensuing investigation opens up a host of other stressors for both First Responders and victims, potentially altering their lives in ways they often cannot understand. Just one very difficult case and a protracted investigation adds to the already heavy workloads being carried by investigators and exacerbates the chronic stress that is already part of the job. Similar demands with diminishing resources to meet those demands is an unrelenting burden for all First Responders as they also face critical staff shortages and hiring and retention challenges.

Second, depending on the magnitude and nature of an incident, multiple First Responder agencies often respond to and are needed on the same calls, meaning that practically every call involving serious injury and death will impact law enforcement, fire and EMS. The most difficult calls will continue to reverberate throughout these different First Responder agencies and over time will comprise a shared history that bonds these dedicated public servants to one another.

Third, while most of the public think of law enforcement, EMS and firefighters as the "true" First Responders, there are clearly other highly essential employees working in the public sector who are also subject to similarly high risks of exposure to trauma, both directly and vicariously. Yet they lack the means or tools, commonly available to law enforcement officers, to protect themselves, at least from physical harm. There is no better example than Telecommunicators. Thankfully, some states have passed legislation to recognize Telecommunicators as full-fledged "First Responders" and other states are considering doing so. Over the course of their careers these vital, but often overlooked First Responders will have heard every tragic story imaginable, while working at a console with 911 calls.

Telecommunicators not only provide professional, highly skilled direction and vigilant caring to all those in the field as they are multi-tasking during some of the most horrific incidents. They also have the unenviable burden of being the "first of the First Responders" to experience some of the most harmful sensory exposure over the phone. This exposure includes but is not limited to the sounds of women and children screaming and crying as the Telecommunicator tries to calm and reassure them that help is in route; the ear-ringing sounds of gunshots; pure terror when someone is being assaulted or robbed; hearing someone's last words while they are dying because of an accident or about to kill themselves; remembering the unmistakable sound of the chair, stool or bucket being kicked over before the caller dies by hanging; struggling to make out what is unintelligible while trying to get help to the scene quickly; or hearing the fear and panic in a First Responder's voice who is urgently in route to or already at a scene when he/she is screaming for backup; or worst of all…losing contact with that First Responder who may have wrecked his/her vehicle or been ambushed. For those calls involving a line of duty death (LODD) or line of duty (LOD) injury this level of stress for the Telecommunicator is unbearable and potentially career-ending as it also spills over into his/her personal life, altering his/her worldview where everything can now appear as a crisis or potential crisis. All of this sensory exposure is amplified when you consider that scores of other First Responders from multiple agencies are also monitoring radio traffic and in a highly charged state of alert as these most dreaded incidents unfold. Every day, and often outside the awareness of the public they safeguard, many of these First Responders risk life and limb to race to the aid of a victim or one of their own who is injured or in danger.

Telecommunicators not only provide professional, highly skilled direction and vigilant caring to all those in the field as they are multi-tasking during some of the most horrific incidents. They also have the unenviable burden of being the "first of the First Responders" to experience some of the most harmful sensory exposure over the phone.

Fourth, there are other workgroup populations that could be considered "quasi" First Responders just in terms of the risks that come with their professions. Examples include social workers and public health staff whose work responsibilities make them very front-facing with the public, often taking them into some of the most unsafe neighborhoods where they encounter individuals and families who are heavily exposed to an array of crises and traumatic incidents. Some of these encounters in homes and businesses may be with individuals who can potentially become violent and disruptive toward any public official.

I would consider the Chaplaincy Program probably one of the most critical programs that can be instituted for First Responders in any jurisdiction. The stressors, hatreds, divorces and suicides that are happening among First Responders... especially in today's world are alarming. We need help...we need support, whether we can admit it or not.

Lt. Jerry Hobbs
Retired
Forsyth County Sheriff's Office

First Responders in Forsyth County, North Carolina

There are, by conservative estimates, more than 3,200 First Responders (law enforcement, fire, EMS) personnel serving in Forsyth County, North Carolina.

Since its inception the FRCP has provided and continues to provide on-call mobile crisis intervention services 24 hours/7 days a week/365 days to these public servants.

Additionally, the FRC Team also provides service to the nearly 1,000 non-First Responder employees which comprise over 20 other Forsyth County departments, the largest of which are Public Health and Social Services.

The FRC Team's services are also utilized by five key groups on the Wake Forest University (WFU) campus, primarily the WFU Police Department, whose members are subject to higher levels of critical incident stress and need support that is not readily available through traditional campus resources.

The FRCP's service population is much larger than workforce numbers alone would indicate and essentially quadruples this active employee count, encompassing the family members of First Responders and a growing population of First Responder retirees who routinely request the FRC Team's support. If one assumes as a most conservative estimate that each First Responder (active or retired) has at least two significant other family members, then the size of the "parish" being served by the FRC Team easily equates to 12,000 individuals.

Indeed, this ever-growing population of those for whom FRCP provides services expands exponentially each year, and the FRC Team is often called to respond to incidents in contiguous cities and counties, with whom there is no formal contract. (See the next chapter about the history of the FRCP for more details.)

Local and National Credentialing Bodies and Programs for First Responder Chaplaincy

Most volunteer chaplaincy programs assisting First Responder agencies do not require any specific Clinical Pastoral Education units of training (CPE, the formal chaplaincy training program located in hospitals) or credentialing by the American Clinical Pastoral Education, ACPE (formal national Board for certifying chaplains to work in hospital and other settings). *However, it is clear that the required level of training for these programs has a baseline far below that implemented in our Atrium Health Wake Forest Baptist Health (AHWFB) FRCP.* All AHWFB FRCP staff must be certified through ACPE. In many other cases, clergy volunteers lack any clinical hospital training and some have minimal or no formal theological training.

For this reason, most hospitals, certainly large medical centers, out of appropriate concern for staff, visitor and patient safety, have been and remain understandably skeptical of clergy volunteers, especially those who identify as "chaplains" but lack any clinical training or CPE. In fact, some medical centers are stepping away from using volunteers for spiritual care purposes.

However, it must be noted that most medical centers have either missed or ignored opportunities to expand professional chaplaincy outside the institutional walls. It is for this reason that many disparate volunteer chaplaincy programs came into existence in recent decades to fill a vacuum created by the fact that other longstanding chaplaincy programs were primarily hospital-centric and, like the hospitals in which they reside, these programs, were far too risk-averse to address the vast needs of First Responders and survivors-victims-witnesses of crime and trauma in their respective communities. This institutional-community disconnect with respect to collaboration and networking is especially ironic considering how frequently First Responders of all types and the trauma victims they encounter daily are the primary users of emergency departments across the nation.

So, it is not surprising that one of the responses to this hospital-centric focus of chaplaincy in recent years, is evident in the current plethora of chaplaincy groups and organizations that have sprung up nationally to address what are obvious needs for support with First Responders and their families.

Almost all these disparate chaplaincy groups are comprised of volunteers with little if any stable funding and minimal structure and networking. Most are well-intentioned, quite well-organized and many have earned the trust of their communities. They are to be commended for making a vital difference their respective communities to fill a void of support. But other volunteer chaplaincy organizations espouse various and often conflicting understandings of what defines a chaplain or chaplaincy, appropriate screening and training and chaplaincy's role in increasingly diverse and inclusive communities. Some volunteer chaplaincy groups believe it is sufficient to simply be "called" into the work and complete online classes or attend a few conferences and get a certificate of attendance. More concerning is that some are highly polarized and routinely engage in tactics that any professional chaplain code of ethics would condemn due to the irreparable harm such tactics could inflict upon already traumatized victims, as well as First Responders and the agencies and communities they represent and serve.

A significant amount of the FRCP Director's training over the years with clergy has been enhancing their skill set but also helping them appreciate how their own profession has inadvertently contributed to the revictimization of those already hurting. The Director firmly believes that the FRCP, as a model for specialized chaplaincy, is privileged to be able to address some of these challenges by offering unique training to chaplains but also to local clergy who seek to improve their skills as crisis responders in their respective communities.

For these and other reasons, volunteerism with respect to providing chaplaincy services for First Responders is noble but has inherent disadvantages. This unique form of chaplaincy requires sustainable funding and resources and cannot be scaled using only a volunteer approach.

It has also become increasingly apparent that Employee Assistance Programs (EAPs) and similar programs (that are typically funded by city and county governments as well as the private sector) are woefully inept at addressing the trauma-related needs of First Responders for a variety of reasons, but also the trauma-related needs of their non-First Responder employees and the public. COVID-19 has only underscored this reality as First Responders are under assault by multiple stressors both at home and work.

A significant amount of the FRCP Director's training over the years with clergy has been enhancing their skill set but also helping them appreciate how their own profession has inadvertently contributed to the revictimization of those already hurting.

The FRC Team's primary strength is derived from strong, carefully built webs of trust made possible by being embedded in those First Responder communities it serves.

Both EAPs and strictly voluntary approaches to chaplaincy do not allow for the embedded presence that only full-time staff chaplains can provide. The FRC Team's primary strength is derived from strong, carefully built webs of trust made possible by being embedded in those First Responder communities it serves. The FRC Team's distributive model of remote working, in place even before COVID-19, is a critical part of the program's effectiveness.

It has also not helped to raise the bar of chaplaincy services or educate the public about these services when we still have leaders across the spectrum of First Responder agencies who fail to understand that chaplaincy, especially First Responder chaplaincy, is a specialized ministry and must be differentiated from the roles of traditional clergy and professional chaplains who work in other settings. The most prime examples of this misunderstanding include the common misspelling of "chaplain" as *"chaplin"* and attributing the title "chaplain" to any clergy or layperson serving in some volunteer capacity with a First Responder agency.

It is also noteworthy that a large percentage of volunteer "chaplains" associated with law enforcement have a ministry focused primarily, if not exclusively, on incarcerated populations in jails and prisons, not on First Responders, their family members or on crime and trauma victims in the larger community.

Also, many of these volunteer chaplaincy groups have different protocols, resources and scopes of practice (e.g., railroad chaplains). Additionally, the signature difference with the FRCP is the fact that it is an integral part of a highly diverse health system. For example, AHWFB alone has a workforce of more than 70,000, spanning a footprint of 40 hospitals and 1,400 care locations. Specifically, it is based at a Level One Trauma Center where it represents and serves many community stakeholders. Most other chaplaincy groups are endorsed, affiliated with or supported by an agency or organization that typically serves a narrower population.

National and State Agencies

Some of the most common national credentialing boards for volunteer First Responder chaplaincy include the Federation of Fire Chaplains, International Conference of Police Chaplains (ICPC) and International Fellowship of Chaplains (IFOC).

The Federation of Fire Chaplains was established in 1978 and its training includes 16 hours of basic ministry to firefighters and fire victims, Critical Incident Stress Debriefing (CISD), fire department funerals and fire chaplaincy basics. Their advanced program (with a prerequisite of five years of experience in the field) includes Critical Incident Stress Management (CISM), pastoral crisis intervention, grief counseling and more. The Federation of Fire Chaplains has over 1,500 members and serves the regions of Great Lakes, New England, Mid-Atlantic, Midwest, South Central, Southeast, Southwest and International.

The International Conference of Police Chaplains serves 60 sites across 40 states, including North Carolina (contained in ICPC Region 8) and boasts 2,100+ members. Their training includes 10 contact hours of CEUs, one CPE unite, ICPC Training credits and twelve core courses.

The International Fellowship of Chaplains (ICPC) requires 40 hours of training in domains of death notification, post-traumatic stress disorder, trauma, grief and loss, self-care and more. This body can also certify and ordain members. They serve 32 locations across 18 states. North Carolina sites served include Charlotte (IFOC Metrolina Chaplain Corps), Fayetteville (Sandhills Community Chaplain Corps) and Moravian Falls (Blue Ridge Chaplain Corps).

Concerns of Police Survivors (C.O.P.S.) is a national organization with state chapters serving families of fallen officers. C.O.P.S also hosts annual meetings and camps for the survivors of fallen officers, including spouses, parents, children and peers. Counseling is available at these camps for participants.

History of the Wake Forest Baptist First Responder Chaplaincy Program

The Wake Forest Baptist Health FRCP has its origins in the decades' long work of its Founder and Director, Chaplain Glenn Davis who served for over 27 years (July 1988–April 2016) as the full-time Chaplain and Victim Counselor for the Forsyth County Sheriff's Office (FCSO). Chaplain Davis is both an ordained minister and Clinical Pastoral Education (CPE) trained. He continues to serve as the Chaplain Liaison to the FCSO as the FRCP Director.

During his tenure with the FCSO, Chaplain Davis provided deeply embedded and highly mobile, on-call chaplaincy support and crisis intervention to survivors-victims-witnesses of catastrophic incidents by being "in the trenches" and responding on scene to workplaces, homes, churches and hospitals. He delivered hundreds of death notifications and other traumatic messages and provided bereavement aftercare and referrals to survivor families. Chaplain Davis also responded to critical incidents locally and regionally and led national crisis response teams with NOVA (National Organization for Victim Assistance) to disasters to assist a broad spectrum of First Responders and survivors-victims-witnesses.

Chaplain Davis was able to use his experiences to train and consult with others on a wide array of topics including wellness, community crisis response, Critical Incident Stress Management (CISM), death notification and traumatic grief for many professional groups, including the International Conference of Police Chaplains (ICPC), Winston-Salem/Forsyth County Public Schools, NC Victim Assistance Network (NCVAN), Southern Baptist Convention's Disaster Relief personnel, numerous law enforcement agencies, hospital chaplains, Motorsports/NASCAR chaplains, hospices and ministerial associations.

Chaplain Davis learned after leaving his CPE behind that he was an anomaly in this "outside the hospital walls" community-based, embedded model of mobile crisis chaplaincy. He also had a front row seat at observing how First Responders and their families were routinely exposed to trauma and extended chaplaincy support to them as well. The realization came early that such noble and gratifying work comes with a heavy price and underscored the need for constant self-care. In order to sustain himself, help motivate others toward better self-care and to change the organizational culture, he developed the Wellness Program for the FCSO that is still active and provided wellness education to First Responders as a certified Physical Fitness Instructor for 20 years with the NC Justice Academy.

Given the scope and demands of the on-call work, Chaplain Davis proactively sought out a select group of local clergy who demonstrated some affinity for this specialized ministry and were willing to undergo extensive volunteer training. This led to Chaplain Davis equipping Chaplain Response Teams in Forsyth County but also in other cities/counties to help provide on-scene, post-trauma support to assist First Responders and survivors-victims-witnesses in their respective communities.

See Appendix 3 for a short article about Chaplain Davis's work in the FCSO from the School of Pastoral Care at Wake Forest Baptist.

Interestingly, his family history links him to the risks and sacrifices endured by all First Responders. His paternal grandfather, George A. Davis, was killed in the line of duty (LOD) at the age of 49, on September 2, 1918, in Marion County, SC. Chaplain Davis was able to do the necessary research in 2018 to have his grandfather's line of duty death (LODD) officially documented

Chaplain Davis learned after leaving his CPE behind that he was an anomaly in this "outside the hospital walls" community-based, embedded model of mobile crisis chaplaincy.

In his nearly 28-year career with the FCSO, and prior to that while working under a two-year federal grant, Chaplain Davis responded to a broad range of crises and disasters, often at the request of other agencies, locally, regionally and sometimes nationally with other crisis response teams.

and his name inscribed on the National Law Enforcement Memorial in Washington, D.C., nearly a century after his death.

The National Law Enforcement Officers Memorial is the nation's monument to law enforcement officers who have died in the line of duty. Dedicated on October 15, 1991, the Memorial honors federal, state and local law enforcement officers who have made the ultimate sacrifice for the safety and protection of our nation and its people.

In his nearly 28-year career with the FCSO, and prior to that while working under a two-year federal grant, Chaplain Davis responded to a broad range of crises and disasters, often at the request of other agencies, locally, regionally and sometimes nationally with other crisis response teams. Below describes details of only a fraction of that work.

Grant-funded Years

Prior to Chaplain Davis's extensive career with the FCSO as Chaplain/Victim Counselor he worked under a two-year federal grant through the Governor's Crime Commission that was administered by the Winston-Salem Police Department (WSPD). His office based at Family Services, proved to be an awkward and inefficient arrangement, since calls for service came primarily from the FCSO. While at Family Services, Chaplain Davis was also the only CPE-trained chaplain and only employee on 24-hour call. Equipped with only a pager and a donated, bag-style mobile phone, he would have to drive his personal vehicle to the Family Services office when deployed on an emergency and once there, enter the office and sign out a company vehicle before proceeding to the emergency. At the end of the call, this process was reversed, always adding a minimum of an hour, and sometimes more, to each deployment. Oftentimes he skipped this transition and used his personal vehicle to respond more quickly to emergencies.

Preston Oldham (the Forsyth County Sheriff at the time), the FCSO staff and the Forsyth County Commissioners were convinced by the end of the grant period that the crisis intervention services made available to staff and survivors-victims-witnesses throughout the City and County were valuable enough to fund permanently. Consequently, a Board of Commissioners vote in July of 1988 funded the position with hard money.

When asked by then FC Commissioner John Holleman where Chaplain Davis wanted the program to be housed, his response, though at that time he understood little of local politics, was without hesitation "the FCSO." Having endured the challenges and disillusionment of relying solely on grant funding, he believed that the current Sheriff and future Sheriffs would have the necessary power as elected public servants to effect change and ensure that this vital work would be funded and sustained for many years.

Chaplain Davis's Experience with Regional and National Crisis Response Teams

Numerous crises early in Chaplain Davis's work shaped his ethics and beliefs about First Responder chaplaincy. On Sunday night, July 17, 1988, just weeks after Chaplain Davis officially joined the FCSO as its only Chaplain, Forsyth County experienced one of its worst tragedies. Michael Hayes, experiencing psychotic episode, walked out of his failing moped business, armed with a .22-caliber rifle, and began waving down traffic on Old Salisbury Road near the Forsyth/Davidson County line. Hayes started shooting people who he believed were "demons" as they slowed down at the intersection. When the shooting finally ended, he had murdered four people—Crystal Cantrell, Tom Nicholson, Melinda Hayes and Ronnie Hull—and wounded five others before a FCSO deputy shot and incapacitated him. The injured victims, bereaved families and the entire community were forever scarred by this tragedy, which received national attention and reshaped local politics.[3]

Chaplain Davis's responses to some regional disasters included the tragic deaths of three fans at an Indy car race at Lowes Motor Speedway, May 1, 1999, and the walkway collapse at that same location on March 20, 2000.[4]

Chaplain Davis's deployment to both tragedies noted above stemmed from his having led multiple crisis response training workshops with NASCAR chaplains at Lowes Motor Speedway and at

Chaplain Davis took on the challenge using his personal time/weekends to attend multiple races and embed with NASCAR driver teams in and around the Charlotte/Concord area and other racetracks to learn as much as possible about the culture and the needs, in order to design training that would help the chaplains (and their spouses) who were committed to this racing ministry.

other locations. A few years earlier, Motor Racing Outreach (MRO),[5] a ministry based at Lowes Motor Speedway, had approached what was then known as the School of Pastoral Care at WFBH about seeking trauma-informed training for their "chaplains" who provided ministry at racetracks across the US. They routinely witnessed serious, if not deadly, accidents and injuries that impacted drivers, racing teams and fans. However, they lacked essential crisis intervention skills and a thorough understanding of traumatic grief. Sharon Engebretson, then head of the CPE program at WFBH, referred MRO to Chaplain Davis, explaining that she and other hospital staff at the time lacked the skills, resources and time to provide this type of mobile crisis response training for this unique subset of chaplains working in such an exclusive culture.

Chaplain Davis took on the challenge using his personal time/weekends to attend multiple races and embed with NASCAR driver teams in and around the Charlotte/Concord area and other racetracks to learn as much as possible about the culture and the needs, in order to design training that would help the chaplains (and their spouses) who were committed to this racing ministry.

Also, during this time he met other key persons such as H.A. "Humpy" Wheeler, then President of Lowes Motor Speedway. It was Humpy and his team who asked Chaplain Davis to not only provide crisis interventions for many impacted staff groups after these tragedies but to also personally accompany him when he visited each of the bereaved families whose loved ones died in the May 1999 tragedy.

In that May 1999 accident, a wheel that came off an Indy race car, bounced over a fence and traveled, while spinning at a high rate of speed like a buzz saw, into the spectator seats, instantly killing three fans. Hundreds of nearby spectators were horrified by the scene, the amount of blood and nature of the injuries. Interestingly, thousands of others attending the race on the other side of the large oval track only saw mass chaos and were unaware of the tragedy that was unfolding.

Chaplain Davis's work was further influenced by multiple deployments with the National Organization for Victim Assistance (NOVA), which pioneered the first national community crisis response team (CCRT) model. Those deployments included providing care in the aftermath of the Amtrak train crash in Baltimore County on January 4, 1987 (Amtrak's deadliest crash at the time); the Ole Miss sorority walkathon accident, March 26, 1987, that killed five; the Carrolton, KY, bus crash, May 5, 1988, that killed 27, 24 of whom were children.

Chaplain Davis also deployed with NOVA crisis teams to Hurricane Andrew in Florida in 1993, the Oklahoma City bombing of the Alfred P. Murrah Building on April 19, 1995, to other natural disasters in Mississippi and Kansas, working with firefighters, law enforcement officers, teachers, clergy, funeral directors, parents and others whose lives were forever altered by these tragedies.

The 1988 Carrolton, KY, bus crash[6] was, by far, the worst tragedy that Chaplain Davis ever attended as part of a NOVA crisis response team to the community of Radcliff, KY. It remains the worst drunk-driving tragedy in KY and the US and as such gave much prominence to Mothers Against Drunk Driving (MADD).

Chaplain Davis reported that he would never forget arriving in Radcliff, KY, and seeing a processional of over a dozen identical hearses carrying the bodies of child victims. He met with several groups of parents, teachers, clergy and funeral home directors all of whom needed much support to deal with the magnitude of so many juvenile deaths. The funeral directors also struggled with seeing and handling the hundreds of artifacts (stuffed animals, cards, other mementos, etc.) delivered to the funeral homes to be placed inside and around the small caskets.

The fact that this was a human-induced crime (caused by an impaired driver, Larry Mahoney), and not an accident, added to the intense pain, rage and complicated grief. Chaplain Davis spent significant time at one church where many of the bereaved families attended. While there he witnessed some of the worst revictimization and retraumatization he had ever seen inflicted on grieving families by clergy. This experience compelled him to spend the rest of his career teaching faith leaders and congregations how to be more effective and compassionate caregivers by acknowledging their potential to do further harm to those who are already so wounded and vulnerable.

The 1988 Carrolton, KY, bus crash was, by far, the worst tragedy that Chaplain Davis ever attended as part of a NOVA crisis response team to the community of Radcliff, KY.

Even though the new chaplaincy program would be relocated and anchored at WFBH, the FCSO would remain a primary stakeholder and see its chaplaincy services not only continue uninterrupted but expanded, making the FCSO a key partner in the innovation.

The sensory exposure accompanying this tragedy was extraordinarily graphic and prolonged. Arriving First Responders were powerless and helpless as they watched 27 people (24 of whom were children) burn to death.

While responding to all these community tragedies and continuing to serve as a chaplain for local First Responders, it became increasingly evident to Chaplain Davis that many medical centers had missed opportunities to develop professional chaplaincy outside the hospital walls to engage with, learn from and collaborate with First Responder agencies and all those committed to helping First Responders and their families. As far back as late 1999, when the world was fearing Y2K, Chaplain Davis approached WFBH (where he had completed his CPE) to discuss how a First Responder chaplaincy model (then anchored at the FCSO) might work more effectively at a Level One Trauma Center and benefit multiple agencies and the broader community. The concept was well-received by several colleagues but, as noted previously, much too innovative at the time for the more risk-averse environment of the medical center.

First Responder Chaplaincy Program Moves to Wake Forest Baptist Health

In 2016, WFBH VP of Faith Health, Rev. Dr. Gary Gunderson, recognized Chaplain Davis's outstanding work and wanted to bring the work under FaithHealth at what is now Atrium Health Wake Forest Baptist (AHWFB), but he also wanted to grow the program and train others in the work that Chaplain Davis had so ably done for decades. Sheriff William T. "Bill" Schatzman, who had always fully supported Chaplain Davis's work, embraced this new, ambitious plan. Even though the new chaplaincy program would be relocated and anchored at WFBH, the FCSO would remain a primary stakeholder and see its chaplaincy services not only continue uninterrupted but expanded, making the FCSO a key partner in the innovation. It was Sheriff Schatzman's hope that all law enforcement agencies, as well as other First Responders, would eventually benefit from the FRCP. The program's goals, as the FRC Team grew, included expanding chaplaincy services to the families of First Responders (active and retired) in Forsyth County and the surrounding region, networking with other chaplain and peer support groups and providing education to enhance the resiliency and crisis response skills of local clergy and mental health providers.

The FRCP began on May 19, 2016, by hiring Chaplain Davis as the Director and is an innovative approach to chaplaincy designed to care for our First Responders, our most valuable and vulnerable public servants, while also helping many bereaved families and other survivors-victims-witnesses of traumatic events. The FRCP is hospital-based but community-focused with a strong emphasis on public health and wellness. Anchoring the FRCP inside of a Level One Trauma Center, a daily convergence point for First Responders, also gives it credibility, sustainability and the neutrality so vital to ensuring that the program's services can be available and accessible to all agencies, regardless of staffing or funding resources, rather than "planting" the program in any single agency where it would be more susceptible to politics, turf issues, leadership turnover and unstable funding.

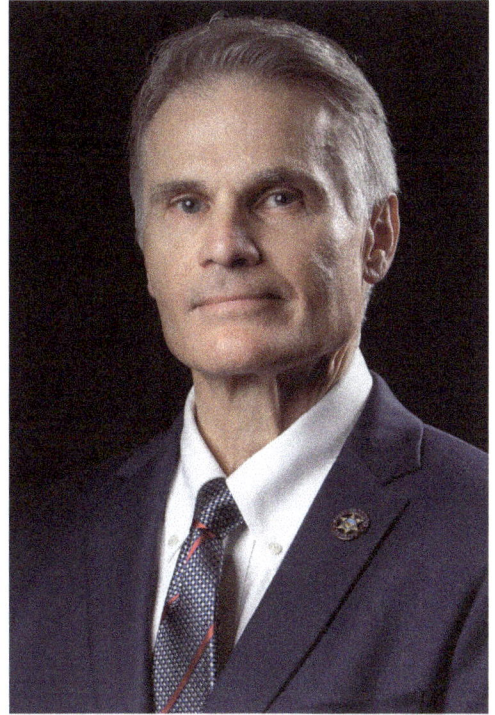

Rev. Glenn Davis, FRCP Founder and Director

Employee Assistance Program (EAP) and FRCP Comparison

As a condition of a 2017 funding ($75,000) provision, Forsyth County designated the FRC Team (not the Employee Assistance Program or EAP) as the primary go to resource for trauma-related needs for ALL county employees, not just First Responders. This change was to specifically address a range of needs that were not being met by the County's EAP provider, with the greatest concern being the need for a highly accessible and immediate mobile crisis on-scene response. Over the past several years, numerous incidents have underscored the reality that any local government employee (or any community resident for that matter), whether at work or at home, can be directly or indirectly affected by trauma, which has the potential to impair work performance and quality of life for that individual as well as his/her family and peers.

Some *actual* scenarios that necessitate a competent, well-planned, immediate and strategic crisis response to individuals and groups are listed below:

- A County employee receives a call from a peer or supervisor informing him/her that another peer, or family member of a peer, or former co-worker, etc. has died (by car accident, suicide, heart attack, drowning, overdose, homicide, etc.) while at home, work or on vacation.

- A client/customer is seriously injured or dies suddenly on work premises (an overdose in a public bathroom, a heart attack in front of numerous witnesses, or an accident in the workplace while operating machinery or in other circumstances).

- A peer or co-worker succumbs to a pre-existing illness such as cancer.

- A peer or co-worker is arrested for or is a victim of domestic violence, or is the victim of or suspect in another crime such as child molestation; embezzlement, etc.

- An employee witnesses a drive-by shooting on the way to/from work.

- The employee witnesses a horrible car accident on the way to or from work or sees a child struck and injured or killed while getting on or off a school bus.

- The employee caused the above accident or was the one who struck and killed the child.

- An employee, along with other witnesses, sees a tree surgeon in their neighborhood be crushed to death while working on an oak tree. His mutilated body is highly visible as children are arriving home from school and firefighters are on the scene recovering his body.

- An employee's normally calm neighborhood near the medical center is suddenly overrun with law enforcement officers after a barricaded subject sets fire to the home and begins discharging a weapon.

Other key differences exist between the County's EAP provider and the FRCP: 1) EAP's inability as a faceless entity to provide a direct means of accessing care; 2) EAP's inability to provide mobile, on-scene crisis intervention services at all hours; and 3) The FRC Team is embedded in the agencies it serves, showing up regularly at critical and non-critical times. The FRC Team also is highly accessible while also building and sustaining webs of trust before crises ever happen that enhance the team's effectiveness.

The FRC Team is embedded in the agencies it serves, showing up regularly at critical and non-critical times. The FRC Team also is highly accessible while also building and sustaining webs of trust before crises ever happen that enhance the team's effectiveness.

The FRC Team, by being embedded and present with employees in their respective work environments, is a highly accessible early intervention resource and can help troubled employees make informed decisions about their care.

EAPs, in some cases, can serve simply as another tool of management, funded by and controlled by management. In such cases, EAPs are not a "human" resource that exists to advocate for individual employees. Many EAPs are not a reliable early intervention resource. Supervisors often turn to EAP as a disciplinary action when employees are in trouble, which sets up an adversarial relationship when employees do not willfully seek out or trust EAP's services. In contrast, the FRC Team, by being embedded and present with employees in their respective work environments, is a highly accessible early intervention resource and can help troubled employees make informed decisions about their care. This therapeutic alliance provides for more immediate intervention by the FRC Team and often leads to quicker resolution. Additionally, the FRC Team, by being embedded in the system but not owned by it, is able to speak truth to power and advocate for the most vulnerable and powerless. See a summary of these differences between EAP and the FRC Team's work in Table 1.

The FRC Team can best ensure its goals are successfully accomplished by obtaining additional staffing and funding to address demonstrated needs. Since the initial contract between WFBMC and the County was signed on August 1, 2017, the FRCP's target population has only grown along with requests for service. The FRC Team continues within its limited resources to respond to calls for service to address crisis-related needs that have, in many cases, traditionally been entrusted to EAP. The level of responsiveness and competence demonstrated by the team, and documented by those who have been helped, has generated other referrals and requests for help. Most importantly, it has cultivated trust across multiple agencies within and outside the County. However, these new encounters and collaborations have increased demand and taxed the FRC's Team's resources. The growing need offers further proof that no other resource entity in the region is providing a sustainable, proactive model of providing mobile, on-call crisis intervention services for First Responders and communities impacted by trauma.

The FRC Team is laser-focused on caring for our most valuable and vulnerable public servants but also the "least of these"

Table 1. Comparison of EAP and the FRCP

Category	Employee Assistance Program (EAP)	First Responder Chaplaincy Program
Cost	Free to employees and household family members	Free to employees and household family members
Service Availability	Phones answered 24/7/365 by live reps who often work remotely and are not known to staff. Appointments available only during regular business hours, often with significant wait time.	Phones answered by chaplains 24/7/365, who are known and trusted by staff. Depending on the severity of the situation, the chaplains will provide on-site, in-person support. County First Responder staff routinely mobilize the chaplains on difficult calls.
When to Call	If feeling stressed or overwhelmed	If you are in crisis, after experiencing trauma directly or vicariously (such as death and/or serious injury, illness), or have had sensory exposure to any critical incident causing distress that is impairing functioning at work or at home
Services Provided	Trained consultants will listen to your issues and connect you with resources. These consultants can help with relationship issues, financial and legal concerns and health care navigation, overall stress, mild anxiety or depression and grief.	Highly trained chaplains who understand your work life and context will respond immediately to requests to assist with your concerns and connect you with resources. Call if you need help with: • Crisis de-escalation • Support for First Responders • Trauma and/or secondary trauma • On-site group crisis intervention (GCI) for peers/co-workers • In-service education related to wellness/resiliency/crisis intervention
Critical Incident Stress Debriefing	EAP counselors will sometimes be deployed for this, but typically charge extra	FRCP Covers this at no extra charge
Relationship with Human Resources (HR)	The local EAP is often perceived by staff as simply an extension of HR management, so that sharing with them might jeopardize job security or status.	FRCP is part of Atrium Health Wake Forest Baptist (AHWFB), has no connection to EAP and is not directly connected to HR.
Navigation to and Connection to Other Services and Resources	The local EAP connects staff to legal, financial, higher acuity counseling or other needed resources listed above.	FRCP is deeply embedded in the local community and offers services that extend far beyond traditional EAP resources to also provide on-scene mobile crisis response with all county employees having direct accessibility to the FRC Team via cell phone and emails, providing spiritual care, including officiating at funerals, weddings, christenings, etc.

This standing alongside requires compassion and empathy…having willful proximity to the pain and suffering of others. The team advocates that all persons are deserving of this exemplary level of care so that they are treated with dignity, respect and integrity.

who are disproportionately the survivors-victims-witnesses of some of life's most horrific events. The team is highly committed to delivering excellent care and service to these individuals who often feel powerless and in need of advocacy. This standing alongside requires compassion and empathy…having willful proximity to the pain and suffering of others. The team advocates that all persons are deserving of this exemplary level of care so that they are treated with dignity, respect and integrity.

In the FRC Team's daily practice, three objectives are key: 1) providing a sense of safety and security, which is critical when individual's lives have been upended and vulnerabilities are exacerbated; 2) ventilation and validation, allowing individuals in crisis the chance to tell their stories and be heard, and finally 3) preparation and prediction, providing practical guidance for immediate next steps concerning what to expect, how to care for self and avoid the potential for revictimization and retraumatization when survivors-victims-witnesses are already wounded on many levels and at risk of further harm.

Additionally, the FRCP, at the request of the County in March 2018, became the sole provider of chaplaincy and crisis intervention services for 20 Volunteer Fire Departments or VFDs (726 personnel) in Forsyth County.

The FRC Team underwent a significant change in January 2019 that added to an already full workload, as all County employees were notified of the FRCP as a "new benefit" to provide trauma-related services to the County. That meant that over 2,000 County employees had direct access to the cell numbers and emails for each member of the FRC Team.

Command level staff and Telecommunicators also have access to the FRC Team's on-call emergency number that is answered 24 hours a day, 7 days a week and 365 days a year (24/7/365). This level of accessibility and responsiveness to deploy quickly anywhere in the County is unprecedented and has accrued trust that has naturally generated more requests for assistance.

Current Target Demographics

Our target demographic served as of 2021 is the over 3,200 First Responders (law enforcement, fire, EMS) personnel in Winston-Salem/Forsyth County, with that total including the above 20 VFDs' 726 personnel in Forsyth County. Additionally, as noted above, the FRC Team's workload expanded to provide care to over 2,000 County employees in late December 2019.

The FRC Team also provides support to the County's law enforcement retirees (numbering approximately 300 in 2021), believing that the care of chaplains does not and should not stop when these individuals leave active service. If one assumes that each retiree has three significant others (often it's many more), then the FRC Team has under its care another "parish" of 1,000 members who also have direct access by cell and email to the entire FRC Team.

Many of these retired public servants feel abruptly cut off from their communities upon retirement in ways similar to military veterans who have left active duty, and they need care now more than ever. Some retirees are physically wounded and injured over the course of their careers, but many more are morally wounded because of cumulative trauma from having attended so many difficult calls along with the grief of having lost many coworkers and friends to natural death, but also line of duty deaths (LODDs). Decades of hypervigilance as a First Responder is also typically accompanied by a lack of self-care (poor sleep quality, insufficient exercise, poor diet, etc.) which exacts a toll on all aspects of health. As a result, many retirees face an array of physical and mental health challenges, as do their families.

Many retirees have also been disenfranchised and isolated after leaving their careers and struggling to adjust to civilian life with a new identity. They have especially found it difficult to reconcile their years of service and understanding of law enforcement work amidst seismic social changes including the current negative public perceptions of law enforcement, calls for police reform and social unrest. COVID-19 exacerbated this sense of isolation on many levels.

Many retirees have also been disenfranchised and isolated after leaving their careers and struggling to adjust to civilian life with a new identity.

Many law enforcement retirees unhesitatingly say that, while they found meaning and felt a sense of calling in their law enforcement career, they would never encourage a younger family member to make that career choice today. Despite having all these needs for support, this unique subset of First Responders is not counted among the County's workforce numbers like their actively serving peers, and are too easily forgotten.

Beginning March 3, 2021, when COVID-19 restrictions blocked the law enforcement retirees from having their monthly in-person gatherings, the FRC Team scheduled monthly Zoom meetings to remain connected to and supportive of the group. Initially these Zoom meetings included some active law enforcement staff members and an agenda by the FCSO but later transitioned to meetings with only the FRC Team due to the sensitive needs expressed by the retirees for spiritual care and support during COVID-19.

The FRC Team's scope continues to expand as the ranks of law enforcement, EMS and the Fire service increase, and as these First Responder agencies become more advanced and diverse.

Almost all traumatic incidents involve a multi-agency response, putting the FRC Team alongside many First Responders representing different agencies, particularly with incidents resulting in death(s). While the First Responder's focus is on providing security, protection and investigative skills on these calls, the FRC Team's focus is on caring for all those traumatized, including bereaved family members, but also those First Responders who are impacted. The FRC Team also utilizes a myriad of resources to work with all NC counties and other states to help deliver traumatic messages, death notifications and provide follow-up care, all of which can be very time-consuming. Additionally, the FRC Team is often tapped to handle other crisis situations (e.g., homicides, assaults, domestic violence) and referrals outside of Forsyth County.

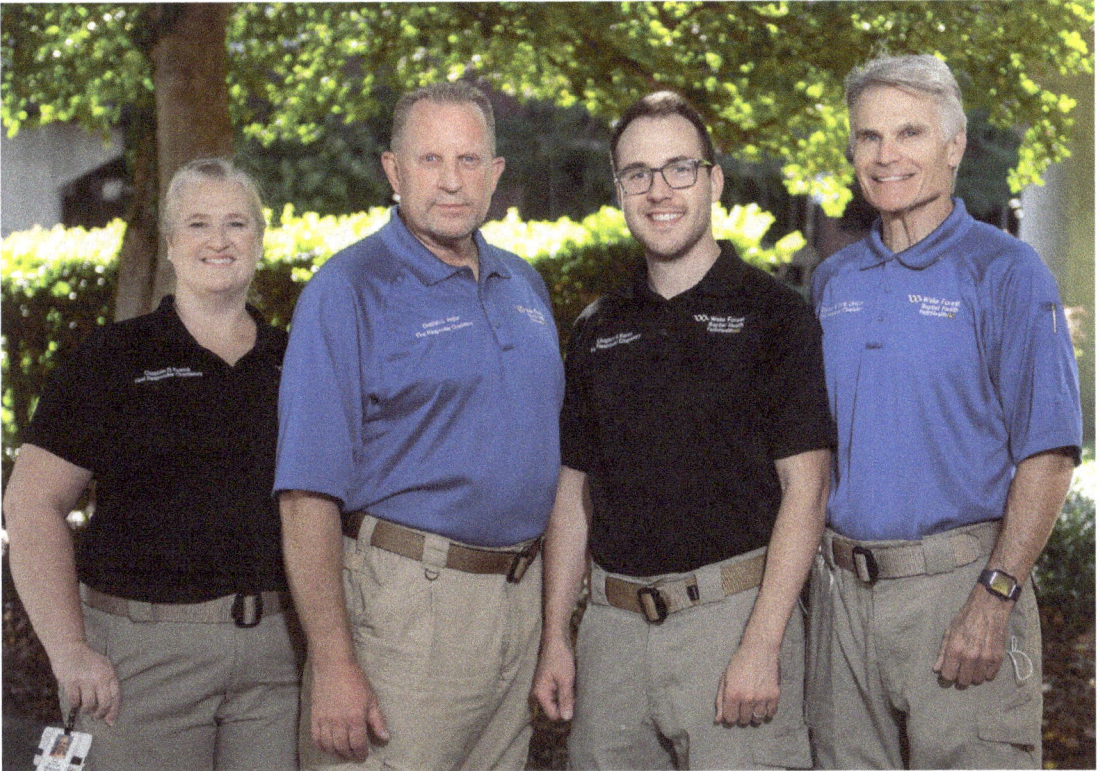

Current FRCP Team, 2021: (left to right) Dana Patrick, Jeff Vogler, Aaron Eaton, Glenn Davis

Mission and Vision of the First Responder Chaplaincy Program

The mission of the FRCP program, using AHWFB as a forward operating base, is highly intentional and proactive with respect to improving health, elevating hope, advancing healing (by teaching wellness, better coping skills, providing grief and post-trauma support and referring as needed) for both First Responders and the community.

The vision of the FRCP entails that everywhere the FRC Team works, it advances health and wellness through collaboration, excellence and is a true innovation within the chaplaincy domain.

Key Features of the First Responder Chaplaincy Program

The FRC Team's connection to its many partner agencies lends credibility, stability, sustainability and the neutrality so vital to ensuring that the program's services can be available and accessible to all agencies, regardless of staffing or funding resources.

The FRCP model is one which can be expanded throughout the AHWFB network, but also adapted by other hospital systems to provide specialized chaplaincy training and expand their services to First Responders and deal with community trauma.

The FRCP, by using clinically trained chaplains, offers some liability protection for First Responder agencies and prevents the irreparable harm that can result from relying on volunteers or other unskilled providers to handle critical assignments such as death notifications. Such tasks must be handled with the utmost care and skill since they pose great risks to the notifier and those individuals and families being notified.

The growing AHWFB network provides an ideal platform to provide pre-incident education and support for First Responder agencies, other hospitals and faith communities throughout the region, especially those agencies and communities with limited resources. A primary goal of the FRCP is to be a regional resource to other communities and medical centers. The FRC Team already provides education to First Responders in surrounding counties and also receives urgent requests from under-resourced counties in the aftermath of critical incidents.

Other key features of the FRCP include the following. The FRCP is an innovation—a new model and specialization within chaplaincy offering advanced training and a new set of competencies to prepare chaplains to operate more effectively both within and outside the hospital walls. Also, the program is community-focused versus hospital-focused and is an investment in public health and wellness by focusing on our most valuable but vulnerable public servants. The FRCP model is one which can be expanded throughout the AHWFB network, but also adapted by other hospital systems to provide specialized chaplaincy training and expand their services to First Responders and deal with community trauma.

Team Structure

The current FRC Team consists of the following members:

Director (one FTE or full time equivalent)
This role oversees all team operations including convening and leading regular team meetings, ongoing team trainings, providing staff supervision, overseeing on-call coverage along with the team's community engagement and

teaching opportunities, assessing and responding to all agency or community crisis intervention requests from within and outside the County, data collection and serving as the team's primary liaison to all First Responder agencies and community partners; providing on-call backup at critical times.

Three Staff Chaplains (three FTEs)

The staff chaplains develop a team on-call schedule and provide on-call coverage 24/7/365 across the County with emergency calls for assistance coming from all First Responder agencies in Winston-Salem/Forsyth County but also other County and City departments. Other organizations, businesses and churches also call upon the FRC Team for crisis response needs and consultation. ALL First Responders in Winston-Salem/Forsyth County have direct, unimpeded access to the entire team's cell numbers and emails, including an FRC Team email, to request confidential support for them and their family members. The FRC Team also provides in-service education to multiple agencies, facilitates GCIs, provides hospital visitation with First Responders and family members, and is embedded in the First Responder agencies providing ongoing staff support, crisis intervention, referrals and follow-up services, regularly submitting documentation. At the time of this book's publication, there are no students or trainees working with the FRCP.

Team Growth

As of 2021, here are the current FTE FRCP staff and their start dates.

- **Director/Founder of FRCP**
  May 2016 to present

- **FRCP Staff Chaplain**
  July 2017 to present (former Resident)

Key roles and functions of the FRC Team include critical incident response, ongoing staff support, education/consultation and community engagement for a growing list of First Responder agencies and other community partners.

- **FRCP Staff Chaplain**
September 2018 to present (former Resident)

- **FRCP Staff Chaplain**
November 2020 to present (former Resident)

Note that the FRC Team plans to hire another FTE Chaplain in 2022 with the specific goal of developing a more inclusive and diverse program.

Key Roles and Functions of the FRCP

Key roles and functions of the FRC Team include critical incident response, ongoing staff support, education/consultation and community engagement for a growing list of First Responder agencies and other community partners.

Critical Incident Response includes on-scene, post-trauma support for a range of victims and First Responder families, death notifications, the delivery of traumatic messages, as well as more formal GCIs for impacted First Responder agencies, churches, other organizations, campus groups and businesses.

Ongoing Staff Support includes individual crisis intervention, hospital visitation at all area hospitals for sick/injured First Responders, grief support for First Responder staff and family members, and a growing First Responder retiree family, in times of transition and loss. The FRC Team also provides referrals to other agencies and longer term follow-up care via calls, emails and other outreach.

Education/Consultation is provided for a variety of groups (First Responder agencies, churches, universities, etc.) and includes crisis response training and pre-incident education on other topics, such as wellness, resiliency and self-care.

Community Engagement is provided via connections with multiple agencies, organizations, faith communities on a continual basis through constant contact with a wide-ranging referral network across Forsyth County and regional counties.

Training and Trainees

This book is not intended to be a training manual, but readers should know that the FRCP's training is intensive and ongoing, and involves a rigorous three-month long onboarding process that includes several education modules and site visits with the FRCP Director/Founder. These are designed to build upon Clinical Pastoral Education (CPE) to equip trainees with the additional skills needed for this specialization within chaplaincy. Critical components of the training include, but are not limited to:

- Learning how to navigate and constantly recalibrate and assess while moving within multiple First Responder agencies each having different protocols, scores of policies and mandated training requirements pertaining to access, security and internal operations.

- Mastering technology, critical software applications and communication methods to operate effectively and remotely with the FRC Team while adapting quickly to multiple environments.

- Building relationships with hundreds of frontline First Responder and civilian personnel in different First Responder agencies, all having complex and evolving organizational structures.

- Understanding the vast differences between on-call coverage in a hospital-based chaplaincy environment versus in a community-based First Responder model of chaplaincy to a broad coverage area, throughout Forsyth County and, as needed, regional counties.

- Managing heavy, sometimes noxious and often graphic sensory exposure unique to First Responder cultures.

- Contending with many other adverse factors unique to trauma scenes including but not limited to weather, travel, biohazards, secondhand tobacco smoke, risks of emotional/physical injuries, chaos and other challenges of delivering care in unconventional and unfamiliar settings.

This book is not intended to be a training manual, but readers should know that the FRCP's training is intensive and ongoing, and involves a rigorous three-month long onboarding process that includes several education modules and site visits with the FRCP Director/Founder.

- Understanding how to deliver traumatic messages and death notifications (not typical duties of a hospital-based chaplain), while being mindful of the potential for irreparable harm to multiple individuals, families and the FRCP itself, that could result from incompetence or failing to respond.

- Developing effective ways of documenting, tracking, archiving and reporting a variety of interactions and accessing highly sensitive information, while being deployed to a variety of settings.

- Maintaining "fitness for duty" and self-care to counter numerous stressors inherent in First Responder chaplaincy and to mentor others to foster wellness cultures within First Responder agencies.

- Developing disciplined, efficient writing skills for reflection papers and after-action reports regarding crisis calls and GCIs.

Trainee History

In 2017, the Director began formulating and refining ways to bring new chaplain residents and fellows into the FRCP. The Director was opposed to adding students who were merely curious about the FRCP or uncommitted, since this proved to be unfair to the student and did not advance the FRC Team's primary need for full-time staff. Fast-tracking the onboarding or the trust-building processes across multiple First Responder cultures is also not an effective way to scale the FRCP model. Similarly, fast-tracking training also can be costly for the First Responder agencies being served in terms of liability and risks of irreparable harm to the communities they serve.

The first (and only) Chaplain Resident for the FRCP served from August 2018 to January 2019, before departing after a few months for another position. The Director was reminded by this experience that Chaplain Residents must master some critical competencies and onboarding tasks to succeed in the program described earlier to work as a First Responder chaplain.

The first and only FRCP Chaplain Fellow worked from April 2019 to October 2020, after completing a full first-year residency. Unfortunately, her fellowship experience was restrained by COVID-19 restrictions. Addtionally, the FRC Team's work during this period was greatly impacted by the murder of George Floyd, Jr. and subsequent violence and diminished public support for law enforcement in the summer of 2020.

Learning from Training a Resident Still Engaged in CPE

The onboarding process for a resident while still engaged in CPE training was handicapped by the resident's inability to be on-call and deploy immediately with the same dependability as the FRC Team. This limitation along with the amount of direct supervision needed to protect the resident and the integrity of the program, created liability risks for all concerned and made using a resident staffing model to scale the FRCP very challenging.

Based upon this experience, Chaplain Davis determined that it was far less effective and efficient to train Chaplain residents, versus training Chaplain Fellows for the program. Below are general observations about the first Fellowship experience.

Learning from Adding the First FRCP Fellow

Utilizing a Fellow assigned almost exclusively to the FRCP helped to disentangle the student from CPE. However, once onboarding was complete and the Fellow was deemed ready to enter the FRC Team's on-call rotation, a quarter of the year had passed. Learning to navigate the various First Responder agencies and become familiar with all the FRC Team's community partners and protocols largely consumed the rest of the year. So, the Fellow staffing model, though more effective than using a Chaplain Resident still tethered to the hospital, was a very valuable training opportunity for the Fellow, but it came with a high opportunity cost for scaling the FRCP and growing the FRC Team.

The experiences of using both a Resident and a Fellow also provided other key insights that were helpful to refine the training modules for the FRCP. Here are a few examples:

Based upon this experience, Chaplain Davis determined that it was far less effective and efficient to train Chaplain residents, versus training Chaplain Fellows for the program.

1. It is critical for would-be First Responder chaplains to possess the right attributes and temperament to work in highly specialized settings like law enforcement and emergency services. These agencies typically function to a great extent as paramilitary organizations, but it does not follow that candidates for First Responder chaplaincy should be recruited from these or similar fields. It is far more important to identify individuals who have the skill sets and competencies to be embedded in First Responder cultures and maintain role clarity essential to function as chaplains. In other words, it can be very counterproductive to have individuals with former First Responder or military experience serving in the role of chaplain in these settings who cannot or will not respect these distinct boundaries. Many of the critical skills needed by a First Responder chaplain (empathy, active supportive listening, high tolerance of ambiguity, "being with" presence, process-focused) are quite different from the highly reactive, problem-solving, mission-focused, compliance-rewarding skills that are common and essential for First Responders.

2. The onboarding process is intense and challenging. A First Responder chaplain's terrain or mission field encompasses multiple agencies and community partners. Callouts or deployments at the time of a critical incident (death or any other emergency at any hour) could be to any location, including sometimes outside of Forsyth County to deliver a traumatic message or provide post-trauma support to a bereaved family, First Responder or a First Responder's family. Numerous adverse elements and risks (ranging from inclement weather, concerns for physical safety and isolation to name just a few) immediately materialize when a First Responder chaplain is activated and expected to respond expeditiously and show up demonstrating a high degree of competence and crisis management skills at the scene of horrific events within such a large area and alongside scores of impacted survivors-victims-witnesses and First Responders who also have been mobilized.

3. In addition, the technology learning curve is steep and ever-changing. This includes the obvious tools such as laptops and iPhones but a high level of proficiency in needed to safely access and utilize sensitive information and databases in times of emergency, while learning other software networking applications and databases. In addition, compliance with security protocols is required not just at AHWFB but with all the FRC Team's law enforcement partner agencies. Because the FRC Team operates using a distributive, remote model, it is heavily reliant on secure technology and rapid communications. This is also critical for data sharing and storage so that each FRC Team member can function effectively from any remote location without having to be dependent on a physical office or routine office hours. The capacity to deploy quickly as individuals or "swarm" as a team to an incident must be maintained and practiced.

The capacity to deploy quickly as individuals or "swarm" as a team to an incident must be maintained and practiced.

Key Goals in Supporting First Responder Staff

1. Creating a culture of empathy by promoting wellness and resiliency through in-service training to promote individual and organizational health.

2. Providing crisis intervention as needed for both Line of Duty (LOD) and non-LOD crises that impact First Responder families.

3. Hospital visitation for sick and injured First Responder staff and their families, as well as First Responder retirees.

4. Providing support and guidance to First Responder staff and their families in times of bereavement related to death but also other losses and transitions.

5. Facilitating GCIs in the aftermath of critical incidents.

6. Making referrals for a range of personal and family issues when more specialized resources are needed (such as marriage counseling, divorce recovery, financial counseling, etc.).

Though it is called the "First Responder Chaplaincy Program," the scope of the team's work includes the large populations across the spectrum of Forsyth County with whom First Responders interact regularly because of a traumatic event (death, serious injuries, crimes, other catastrophes) who are dealing with multiple forms of grief and loss.

7. Attending and participating, when possible, in the funerals of active or retired First Responder staff.

8. Attending agency-sponsored meetings, ceremonies, and other special celebratory events to provide support.

9. Serving as a liaison between all First Responder agencies and diverse faith groups to help build an inclusive community that values First Responders and their families, as well as contributes to making Winston-Salem and Forsyth County a safe and welcoming place to live.

Learning and Best Practices of the FRCP

The FRC Team has consistently received validation for the quality of its services and as an innovative approach to helping not only all our public servants but also many others in our community and region who are impacted by traumatic events. Though it is called the "First Responder Chaplaincy Program," the scope of the team's work includes the large populations across the spectrum of Forsyth County with whom First Responders interact regularly because of a traumatic event (death, serious injuries, crimes, other catastrophes) who are dealing with multiple forms of grief and loss.

It is essential to note that the potential magnitude of one major incident can result in scores of individuals who comprise these impacted communities of survivors-victims-witnesses. This is true in our neighborhoods, communities, workplaces, churches and schools, but also within our First Responder agencies where a single LOD tragedy, certainly a LODD, regardless of the mode of death, has significant repercussions for the entire agency and the community it serves.

The graphic below illustrates how one crisis event can reverberate throughout a community and entire region to impact not just First Responders but a wide-ranging demographic. It can also be a useful reference when doing a tabletop exercise or an after-action review but, more importantly, it can be a valuable tool for helping chaplains and all care providers better understand the need to constantly hone their crisis response readiness.

The innermost concentric circle can be viewed as the epicenter of the crisis, whether natural or human-induced. For the sake of example, if the crisis is a school or workplace shooting, then waves of First Responders, depending on the magnitude of the crisis (numbers of dead and/or injured, protracted nature of the crisis) arrive to neutralize the threat (if one still exists), provide security and medical intervention.

Many survivors-victims-witnesses can be at or near the epicenter, significantly amplifying the needs and chaos. The other concentric circles show how the crisis quickly becomes multi-layered in terms of expanding emotional impact, numbers of involved individuals and a growing network of affiliated groups linked directly or indirectly to the crisis itself and to the victims and First Responders. While there are only six circles in the graphic, the impact of the crisis on the multiple communities affected by it is often highly diffuse and not defined by the physical location of the crisis event. Similarly, all those impacted have their own subjective experience to the crisis event.

The graphic can be especially helpful for First Responder chaplains to better understand the dynamics of any crisis or disaster, particularly regarding how to assess the impact and potential protracted nature of the crisis, the degree of sensory exposure (based on proximity, duration, intensity and type) and also help with triaging post-trauma support to the most vulnerable individuals and groups.

It is quite common to underestimate the number of individuals who experience some level of trauma either directly or vicariously due to proximity of other factors such as their relationships to other victims and recurring media coverage. Others who have experienced prior trauma or a similar loss or who simply lack adequate coping skills are highly susceptible to any "triggers" associated with the crisis that have the potential to dredge up unresolved grief and past trauma. One of the tasks of the First Responder chaplain is to be vigilant in recognizing this widespread impact and proactive in providing care to this much more nebulous group of individuals, whom the Director calls the "unidentified bereaved."

One of the tasks of the First Responder chaplain is to be vigilant in recognizing this widespread impact and proactive in providing care to this much more nebulous group of individuals, whom the Director calls the "unidentified bereaved."

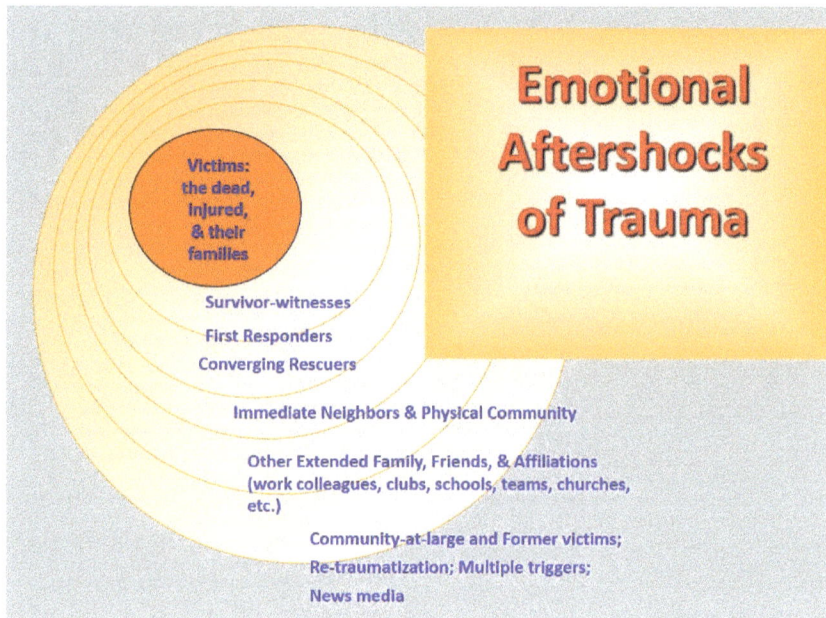

Emotional Aftershocks of Trauma

Victims: the dead, injured, & their families

Survivor-witnesses

First Responders

Converging Rescuers

Immediate Neighbors & Physical Community

Other Extended Family, Friends, & Affiliations (work colleagues, clubs, schools, teams, churches, etc.)

Community-at-large and Former victims; Re-traumatization; Multiple triggers; News media

Because of the FRC Team's responsiveness to these kinds of crises, the number of requests for the team's services only continues to grow and demonstrates the impact of the program's effectiveness within and also beyond Forsyth County. These requests are increasingly coming from organizations who need and value the FRC Team's services but who also report lacking sufficient resources to address their needs, yet they also have no formal agreement with the FRCP establishing protocols or funding for this purpose (e.g., other hospital systems, regional law enforcement agencies, regional 911 centers, private ambulance services, churches in surrounding counties, local banks, other businesses and schools).

Many of these agencies and organizations are appropriately concerned about their lack of crisis preparedness and limited capacity to cope with a critical incident and are interested in pre-incident education to increase crisis response competencies and help bolster the resiliency of their staff when traumatic events occur. However, many other requests are exigent in nature following a life-altering critical incident that has affected multiple staff members who need immediate on-scene help. In such cases, the requesting organizations report that their existing staff support resources (EAP resources or others), if they have them at all, are either non-existent, unavailable, or ill-equipped to respond effectively or expeditiously when traumatic incidents occur. Given the high volume of requests and the refusal to say "no" to incoming requests for help, the Director has found that some agencies are amenable to a "fee for service" agreement in which they can prioritize their needs for chaplaincy services, ranging from high acuity critical on-scene crisis response to in-service education to develop a wellness culture that is more resistant to the impact of critical incidents and chronic stress.

It is important to know that someone who understands, cares about what you have seen and done. It's not normal for anyone to pick up pieces and parts of a body and put it in a bag. It's not normal to see a child eviscerated on an autopsy table. At the end of the day, we end up at home like everyone else eating dinner even though we have seen and done things that just aren't normal. We have to have each other's backs. You can't unburden these things with your spouses and loved ones because of confidentiality. I know first-hand how important it was to have a Chaplain on staff at the Sheriff's Office. You have to be a First Responder, but you are also human. You also have to remind yourself sometimes that you are human and not a work machine.

Sean Reid
Medicolegal Death Investigator
Atrium Health Wake Forest Baptist (AHWFB)

Dealing with FRC Team Members' Vicarious Trauma

The case studies described below all underscore that First Responders and the FRC Team absorb and deal with heavy sensory exposure on some difficult calls, due to the nature of First Responder work. This sensory exposure certainly includes being in the presence of a wide range of grief reactions from survivors-victims-witnesses at various scenes but also includes at times seeing deceased individuals who, depending on the mode of death, can be mutilated, disfigured or in varied states of decomposition. Even if individual team members don't directly absorb these images they are routinely with First Responders who need to process their exposure to these images with the FRC Team.

Self-care and maintenance for the team involves frequent team debriefings, which are invaluable to discuss the most difficult aspects of some crisis calls and potential triggers that might make resolution for the chaplains more difficult. As is true with the First Responders, the FRC Team also finds it more difficult to deal with cases involving serious injury and death among the most vulnerable groups such as children, the elderly and special needs populations. Individual team members also utilize different modalities for coping and are encouraged to continue enhancing their self-care toolbox. Some find it helpful to share generalities of cases with a trusted loved one (while not betraying confidentiality), while also utilizing resiliency skills and spiritual practices such as meditation that served them well in their prior chaplaincy training and roles.

A significant component of the onboarding process for all the staff chaplains is spent carefully preparing them for some of the graphic content they will invariably experience as First Responder chaplains that is potentially far more traumatic than what might be experienced in more conventional chaplaincy settings. Additionally, writing incident after-action reports accomplishes multiple goals of archiving the team's work but also captures insights and challenges, while serving as a tool for reflection with the Director and fellow team members.

Holding and Nurturing Trust

The measurable growth of the FRCP and its effectiveness are in large part a direct result of accruing trust by consistently meeting the FRC Team's goals and commitments to maintain an embedded presence and be highly accessible and responsive to all those the team serves. The FRC Team is intentionally integrated into the workplace cultures of its community partners. This involves the team's on-scene response to deaths and other tragedies but also its presence at non-critical events such as new hire orientations, Command Staff meetings, in-service trainings, promotional events and many other encounters. The team's presence in these non-critical settings makes possible the rapid connections and interventions needed when critical incidents do occur. Additionally, it is the Director's goal that all these integral, embedded relationships are defined in and protected by each respective agency's Standard Operating Procedures (SOP) and/or General Orders. Within any para-military organization, this well-established linkage of the hospital-based FRCP in these non-critical settings strengthens the credibility of the program and conveys to all First Responders and other community partners that the FRCP has clear, policy-defined objectives designed to help them and their families.

The FRC Team often deploys multiple members to some critical incidents as well as to some public events such as trainings and new hire orientations, which offer rich trust-building opportunities. The chaplains are never "off" in a traditional sense. Like First Responders everywhere, the capability to respond quickly when requested by any First Responders' agency's chain of command (COC) from any location is always a possibility. Similarly, the FRC Team understands the potential for an "all hands on deck" call, which might be a LODD or serious LOD injury involving any First Responder. However, there are countless other examples such as any mass casualty event, school shooting or natural disaster that could impact the community, necessitating a large-scale, multi-agency mobilization.

No matter what the need or scale of the critical incident, each expeditious response by the FRC Team is an opportunity to accrue and sustain the trust of our public servants. Each crisis

No matter what the need or scale of the critical incident, each expeditious response by the FRC Team is an opportunity to accrue and sustain the trust of our public servants.

Operationally, the FRC Team practices what is best defined as a highly vigilant, highly mobile and proactive "Search and Find" model of helping versus a reactive model.

call, whether it is manageable by phone or requires a deployment, quickly evolves into a series of important notifications, connections and follow-up even after the crisis abates.

The FRC Team also has the capability of receiving multiple forms of communications in real time as traumatic incidents are unfolding. These methods include, but are not limited to, CAD (computer-assisted dispatch) group messages, initiated by Telecommunicators as well as direct phone calls to the team's emergency on-call number, 24/7 text messaging and phone calls from any First Responder or First Responder family member, as well as direct calls from any First Responder supervisor or other on-scene personnel requesting chaplaincy services to assist staff or survivors-victims-witnesses.

Operationally, the FRC Team practices what is best defined as a highly vigilant, highly mobile and proactive "Search and Find" model of helping versus a reactive model. The team is very committed to providing interventions at the earliest possible stage and expediting help within a critical window of opportunity that can close quickly. This is a radically different method of service delivery from a reactive "Wait and Treat" stationary, non-deployable model that waits for the person in crisis to manifest symptoms and seek help that is rarely immediately accessible or even available. Any delay in receiving help can be further exacerbated when the individual in crisis must navigate a maze of obstacles in the process or have difficulty simply making a human connection such as when they call an 800 number and get voicemail. Early intervention and establishing a therapeutic alliance are especially critical for First Responders, who, in order to do their jobs well, are trained to be skeptical and distrustful to keep themselves and us safe. The FRC Team understands and respects this learned, essential trait and is designed to bring help directly to First Responders in order to deescalate the crisis and alleviate distress at the point of need, making referrals when needed, providing follow-up care and, most importantly, minimizing the stigma of seeking help and protecting confidentiality.

This Search and Find model was a keystone to the Director's earlier work and remains so for FRC Team's work along with constantly building, earning and sustaining trust. This proactive model also includes a high degree of accessibility and responsiveness. This is especially critical considering that one of the most important metrics for measuring success in all First Responder agencies is "response time"…the efficient processing of information and arriving at the point of need, competent and prepared to bring resolution as soon as possible. Since the FRC Team is embedded in the First Responder cultures it strives to adhere to that same high standard of service delivery. A call going unanswered or sitting in a voicemail box or a delayed reaction/response to a request is considered "mission failure" and is unacceptable to the FRC Team. First Responders act with immediacy and expect those alongside them to do the same, especially when they, the First Responders, are the ones needing help.

This reality also sheds some light on why some of the well-intentioned appeals or admonishments First Responders receive from mental health providers are inapplicable or even laughable. When they are "on" it is full mode hypervigilance. The mindful pauses, respites or digital detoxes that the public might leisurely enjoy at any time, and particularly remote work options during COVID-19, have never been options for First Responders. Even when not on active duty, most First Responders maintain their vigilant watch when the public's guards are down. It's a bit ironic that since our ability to live, work and sleep in peace requires the hypervigilance of all First Responders, that some care providers want them to chill. Many will admit that they know full well what they signed up for and are resigned to the fact that few people outside their ranks really understand them or have the intestinal fortitude and courage to do their jobs.

The vigilance and mobility inherent within the FRC Team's "Search and Find" model, that uses embedded clinically trained chaplains with security clearances, enhances the team's effectiveness, giving it unprecedented access to be alongside First Responders within their respective agencies but also in the field. The FRC Team is also proficient in providing continuity of care for those First Responders, who, as a result of LOD injuries or illness, can become patients at any of our local hospitals.

A call going unanswered or sitting in a voicemail box or a delayed reaction/ response to a request is considered "mission failure" and is unacceptable to the FRC Team. First Responders act with immediacy and expect those alongside them to do the same, especially when they, the First Responders, are the ones needing help.

First responder agency heads can attest that the FRC Team's proactive model of crisis intervention that intensely focuses on high quality care for staff has altered the culture of their agencies by promoting individual and organizational wellness and resiliency. As just one example, the team conducts wellness classes for Forsyth County's Volunteer Fire Depts. and EMS.

Wellness and resiliency are critical topics since many First Responders face a perfect storm in terms of being predisposed to many personal and job-related stressors and challenges that impact their physical and mental health. These include working multiple jobs, sleep deprivation from shiftwork along with poor dietary and exercise habits. Considering the many tragic preventable deaths of First Responders caused by COVID-19, life-

One Easter Sunday at about 7:00 AM, I got a phone call from an employee that I supervised. Her brother had just been killed in a plane crash. I consoled her the best I could. Then I called Glenn Davis. BAM, he sprang into action. Getting this woman much needed attention that she needed. It was immediate. Not the next day. IMMEDIATE....

I have a dear friend of 35+ years that was in the hospital with COVID-19. His spirit was broken. No one could go see him and at times he wasn't texting or answering the phone. I emailed the chaplains ... BAM ... I get a phone call from Dana Patrick. She understood that my friend wasn't a Sheriff. It didn't matter. She knew I was worried and therefore she knew she had to act and did she ever. She called my friend twice, letting me know each time that he was hanging in there the best he could. She was also praying for him....

When my grandson was born in Greensboro, N.C and was 2 days old, he had to go to Brenner's with a high fever. I met my wife and daughter there. When the little guy needed a spinal tap, I called Glenn Davis ... BAM ... he showed up moments later. Not hours. Moments. He hugged me in the hallway then came into the room and prayed with my daughter, wife and I. It didn't stop there. Aaron Eaton also came by and prayed with us. Weeks after that, Aaron was coming by my office to make sure the little man was doing well....

style-related diseases (diabetes, obesity, cardiovascular illnesses), all manageable if not preventable in many cases, have remained the top causes of poor quality of life and premature death for all First Responders.

The evidence is clear that safeguarding and investing in the well-being of our First Responders is also an investment in the public health of the communities they serve and protect. The success of this innovative, embedded and proactive approach to providing crisis intervention services to First Responders is, as cited previously, predicated on trust-building. First Responders across multiple agencies consistently report their skepticism and distrust of care providers who do not understand them or the unique stressors impacting them and their families. This gap of trust and

These are just a few examples of probably countless times these chaplains have stepped up in much needed situations. They are more than just a resource. They care. They are friends. They are a shoulder to cry on or a smile when you need it most....

When my wife and I were going to be married, the only name that came to mind was Glenn Davis. It was both of our second marriages and we wanted something small. Eloping basically. Glenn met with us a few times for some pre-marriage counseling and in the end, we were married in our own living room wearing shorts and flip-flops. We were the luckiest couple on the planet. Not only were we getting married, but we were going to be forever tied to Glenn as well, something that means so much more to us than anyone will ever know.

It doesn't matter where I am or what I am doing. If Glenn Davis, Dana Patrick, Aaron Eaton or Jeff Vogler and I make eye contact, there is always time for a quick chat. It doesn't matter what the conversation is. Sometimes they can see when someone is troubled and know they need an ear.

They are all nothing short of amazing.

Sergeant Roger Dunlap
Forsyth County Sheriff's Office

This disconnect, or failure to connect at all, is often perceived as additional harm and can lead to more emotional callouses, fears of more stigma, escalating stress, deteriorating trust and hope, prolonged delays in getting much needed help and a reluctance to seeking help in the future.

misunderstanding quickly becomes apparent when the First Responders who have experienced a critical incident involving intense levels of sensory exposure find that this factor alone often incapacitates the care provider who is traumatized by secondary exposure. This disconnect, or failure to connect at all, is often perceived as additional harm and can lead to more emotional callouses, fears of more stigma, escalating stress, deteriorating trust and hope, prolonged delays in getting much needed help and a reluctance to seeking help in the future.

Multi-Layered and Complex Nature of FRCP

The Director defines First Responder chaplaincy as a parish, or more accurately several mega-churches, without walls and the FRC Team as the ministry staff tending to a growing and constantly mobile extended family of First Responders with ever-evolving needs across multiple agencies. This level of meticulous pastoral care requires a high level of access to ever-changing databases and emergency contact information as staff members are reassigned for a variety of different reasons within and between agencies while others retire from active service. The FRC Team tracks and follows these individuals as they move to different assignments, even beyond retirement, always carefully updating critical information to be able to find and support First Responders but also their significant others very quickly when crises occur. Being able to access any or all this information remotely from any location and transmit highly sensitive information between the team members in the heat of a crisis is essential when a rapid response is needed.

Safeguarding the sensitivity of these interactions and protecting confidentiality are paramount concerns. While some volunteer chaplains may be attracted to the public aspect of this work, it is important to note that much of the FRC Team's activity, outside of providing trainings with groups, is highly covert in nature and the team must be relentlessly overprotective with how it interacts with those who protect us. One misstep, including something as simple as printing a sensitive document, leaving a screen viewable to others, using the phone or joining virtual meetings in settings that lack privacy or moving a confidential document or email from a work account to a personal account could do irreparable harm in terms of damaging hard-earned trust and even be fatal for the FRCP.

> **There has been a lot of negativity** involving law enforcement for a while now and the Chaplains attending some meetings offering devotion and prayers has helped keep our minds and spirits where they need to be. It is amazing how sometimes they say just what you need to hear, just when you need to hear it.
>
> **Sergeant Lori Wood**
> *Forsyth County Law Enforcement Detention Center*

Current Events' Impact

Separating the work of First Responders from current events and stressors is impossible. Election cycles (especially divisive ones), all episodes of gun violence, social unrest, natural disasters and the COVID-19 pandemic are just a few examples that have profoundly impacted the lives and work of all First Responders across the nation since 2020.

The Impact of COVID-19 as an Additional Stressor

First Responders, particularly veteran First Responders, have witnessed firsthand a broad range of critical incidents and disasters (both natural and human-induced or technological), ranging from mass shootings, horrific accidents, terrorist threats, gruesome homicides/suicides, torture, child abuse to sexual assaults, but all of these types of incidents came with some sense of resolution or closure that enabled some degree of compartmentalization. However, unlike all of the above, COVID-19 remains a protracted critical incident, that continues to drain coping resources and exacerbate all other stressors.

Murder of George Floyd in 2020 and Similar Officer Involved Shooting Tragedies

These tragedies have had an immeasurable, ongoing impact and continue to influence the national conversation around police reform.

Some positive results and dialogue have emerged to give hope, but in too many communities the polarization and disconnection between the citizens and those charged to "protect and serve" have only grown, as evidenced by a "circling of the wagons" and entrenchment mindset best known as the "Ferguson Effect" (after the August 14, 2014, police shooting death of Michael Brown, Jr. in Ferguson, Missouri).

Never has there been a greater need for brave, creative leadership among our public servants with these seismic shifts occurring. Agencies are also struggling with hiring and retention issues along with a hemorrhaging of seasoned veteran staff who are retiring or resigning due to growing job-related stressors, a phenomenon well documented in both the public and private sectors as the "Great Resignation" or "Great Quit." These combined factors create a national public safety concern as major staff shortages immediately generate liabilities, just one of which is leaving very young supervisors and less experienced staff on the streets and in detention centers responsible for some of the most dangerous but important work.

Case Studies

Seeing that he had a weapon, she immediately called 911 though he demanded she not do so. With the 911 call still active, he fatally shot himself in her presence.

Note: Narratives of case studies are followed by lessons learned. Also, at the end of each case study are hours/encounter numbers, benchmarked to monetize and better value the exceptional work of the FRC Team.

Case Study #1: Completed Suicide Involving a Retired Law Enforcement Officer (LEO)

The on-call chaplain was dispatched by Telecommunications to respond to a suicide on a weekend afternoon.

Upon arrival, the chaplain spoke to the wife of the decedent and immediately learned that the couple had been experiencing significant stress. It was determined that two adult children, one of whom was out-of-state, had been notified and were also in need of support.

On the day of the suicide, the decedent had urged his estranged wife to return home. When she did so, she found him waiting in the yard for her to arrive. Seeing that he had a weapon, she immediately called 911 though he demanded she not do so. With the 911 call still active, he fatally shot himself in her presence.

The chaplain's goal was one of accompaniment, not to "get her in a good place" but just to walk alongside her and talk with her when she was ready to do so.

The next day, as a part of routine follow-up, the chaplain learned that the Telecommunicator who handled this horrific call personally knew the deceased retiree and also needed support. The chaplain relayed this need to another FRC Team member to expedite care to this Telecommunicator.

A chaplain followed up with the decedent's wife the next day and facilitated arranging a healing conversation between the wife and the Telecommunicator. The wife was grateful that the Telecommunicator had very likely saved her life by getting her to heed the Telecommunicator's advice when the wife was on scene. The trust established between the FRC Team and this one Telecommunicator on this particular call opened up other lines of support and trust for all the Telecommunications staff. In the

Case Study #1: Completed Suicide Involving a Retired Law Enforcement Officer (LEO)

Case Study #1 Suicide	Type of Contact or Incident	# Contacts	Hours Committed by FRCP Team	Initiating Dept.	Other Agencies Involved	Acuity Level of Service for Chaplain	Estimated $ Value, Based on Hours
Day of Event	Crisis Call	Wife, sons (2)	6	FCSO	EMS	Very High	6 hours @ $125 per hour = $750
Day after Event	Support	Dispatcher (2)	4	FCSO Communications	—	Very High	4 hours @ $125 per hour = $500
Week after Event	Support	Wife, son (2)	2	—	—	High	2 hours @ $125 per hour = $250
Six months after Event	Follow-up Calls	Wife, sons, dispatcher (4)	1	—		Moderate	2 hour @ $125 per hour = $250
One Year after Event	follow-up Calls	(4)	1	?	?	Low	1 hours @ $125 per hour = $125
TOTAL		14	14	—	—	Median = Very High	$1875

end, the chaplain was able to make appropriate referrals for all family members to help process their trauma.

The chaplain related that the callout/activation to this acute incident and subsequent follow-up meetings totaled approximately eleven hours of very intense in-person encounters with the wife, calls with the Telecommunicator and adult children survivors.

Lessons Learned from Case #1

- A cascade of calls and connections are often generated by every incident, particularly those involving suicide and other violent deaths.

- The FRC Team's high level of commitment to maintaining continuity of care is demonstrated as the entire team is constantly working in tandem to ensure that all those impacted (bereaved family members, neighbors, witnesses and the involved First Responders) receive appropriate care.

- It is noteworthy that this opportunity to provide follow-up care in the larger community is not always possible within conventional chaplaincy settings, where in many cases, patients, family members, staff and even chaplains are unable to have long-term relationships with patients and families after a patient is discharged or dies. However, for First Responder chaplains, these relationships can exist and grow for many years as part of an extended web of multiple relationships with bereaved family members, as well as both active and retired First Responders. This follow-up care arguably prevents the likelihood of more trauma and violence, and generates more referrals but it is hard to monetize and show impact of a suicide or homicide, such as a domestic violence-related death, etc., that did not occur.

A cascade of calls and connections are often generated by every incident, particularly those involving suicide and other violent deaths.

Case Study #2: Missing Person/Suicide

The entire FRC Team was alerted to a missing person report involving an adult with a substance use history and repeated estrangement from family members. Weeks later, a decomposing body was found by citizens who detected an odor when out walking in a wooded area. Cause of death was determined to be suicide by hanging. The on-call chaplain provided appropriate support to the bereaved family and to the First Responders impacted by this protracted investigation and high level of sensory exposure at the death scene. Other FRC Team members reached out to the parent who discovered the body while walking with his children.

Lessons Learned from Case #2

- The protracted nature of a missing person investigation creates many added stressors for family members and consumes much time and resources of the involved First Responder agencies.

- It is not unusual for the FRC Team to be in standby mode for extended periods to do a death notification and provide

Case Study #2: Missing Person and Suicide	Type of Contact or Incident	# Contacts	Hours Committed by FRCP Team	Initiating Dept.	Other Agencies Involved	Acuity Level of Service for Chaplain	Estimated $ Value, Based on Hours
Day of Event	Crisis Call	4	4	FCSO, Family of Deceased		Very High	4 hours @ $125 per hour = $500
Weeks after Event	Support	6	4				4 hours @ $125 per hour = $500
TOTAL						Median = Very High	$1000

post-trauma support to staff and families pending discovery and positive identification of a missing person later found to be deceased.

- This case also underscores that the FRC Team's highly focused mission to identify and locate the next of kin in the most expeditious manner possible once death is confirmed in order to make an in-person notification and provide support and other resources.

- The sensory exposure component, not only for the First Responders but especially for the untrained, innocent bystanders who happened to accidently discover the body in a case such as this, is powerful and life-altering. For this reason, learning how to contend with the graphic nature of First Responder chaplaincy is a critical part of the team's onboarding process and training.

The sensory exposure component, not only for the First Responders but especially for the untrained, innocent bystanders who happened to accidently discover the body in a case such as this, is powerful and life-altering.

Case Study #3: Officer Involved Shooting (OIS)/Line of Duty (LOD) Injury

A very early morning computer-assisted dispatch (CAD) message from Telecommunications alerted the entire FRC Team to an "officer down" incident. A local law enforcement officer (LEO) had been assaulted by a suspect who then shot the officer multiple times before fleeing the scene. The injured officer was transported to the trauma center where he would face multiple surgeries in the ensuing weeks prior to being discharged and recovering at home. All local and state law enforcement agencies in the County were activated in a manhunt that lasted several hours.

Due to the nature of this call and its extensive impact the Director and the on-call chaplain both immediately deployed to assist First Responders in the impacted community focusing specifically on the paramedics and firefighters who were on scene to treat and transport the officer. The other FRC Team members, initially on standby, were deployed in the ensuing days to help conduct multiple group crisis interventions (GCIs) scheduled with several agencies and handle a high volume of follow-up calls and other meetings.

With the exception of line of duty deaths (LODD), a serious LOD injury and officer involved shooting (OIS) ranks among the most powerful critical incidents First Responders face in their careers.

Lessons Learned from Case #3

- With the exception of line of duty deaths (LODD), a serious LOD injury and officer involved shooting (OIS) ranks among the most powerful critical incidents First Responders face in their careers.

- A First Responder LOD injury call such as this officer involved shooting (OIS), immediately mobilized a multi-agency response involving hundreds of personnel, representing law enforcement and emergency services (Fire and EMS).

- The chronic stress generated by such an incident cannot be overstated. From the outset, this was a highly unstable and chaotic experience for all First Responders, as they are laser focused on the status of the injured officer and on neutralizing the threat, which in this case, involved locating and apprehending the perpetrator.

- This critical incident also demonstrated the advantages of social media and community assistance, as well as the use of technology, in locating and apprehending the perpetrator.

- It also highlighted the value of the accrued trust the FRC Team had already earned with all the affected agencies and how this trust granted the team members immediate access to deploy and be of service on scene and at multiple locations post-incident.

- The near death of a LEO always intensely heightens the sense of vulnerability for all First Responders and their leadership. This anxiety reverberates among all First Responder family members and evokes traumatic memories for First Responder retirees as well.

- Additionally, the FRC Team observed that the entire local community where the incident occurred was visibly shaken as residents felt their sense of safety and perceived invulnerability had been shattered.

- The FRC Team had extensive involvement/follow-up with the impacted agency and Command Staff who found this incident to be life-transforming for them personally and for their agency.

- A day after the incident's occurrence, the FRC Team made a personal connection with the injured LEO and his family members at the medical center to assess their needs and augment their support system. Additional mental health resources were also offered, including the Director taking a therapist to the injured LEO's home to expedite the entire family's ability to receive confidential help as needed during the LEO's extended recovery.

Case Study #3: Officer Involved Shooting/Line of Duty (LOD) Injury

Case Study #3: Line of Duty Shooting	Type of Contact or Incident	# Contacts	Hours Committed by FRCP Team	Initiating Dept.	Other Agencies Involved	Acuity Level of Service for Chaplain	Estimated $ Value, Based on Hours
Day of Event	Crisis Call	4	8	FCSO	EMS, Kernersville PD	Very High	8 hours @ $125 per hour = $1000
Day after Event	Support, officer's family	4	3	FCSO		Very High	3 hours @ $125 per hour = $375
Weeks after Event	GCIs	10	8	PD, EMS, Fire, internal detectives		Very High	8 hours @ $200 per hour with 2 FRCP members = $3200
Weeks after Event	Follow-up Visit in Hospital	2	2			Moderate	2 hours @ $125 per hour = $250
Six Months after Event	Follow-up Calls	6	2			Low	2 hours @ $125 per hour = $250
TOTAL		26	23	4	4	Median = Very High	$5075

This incident underscored how an "officer down" call has a uniquely disturbing and lingering impact on Tele-communicators who are "living and seeing" this incident in their mind's eye from start to finish, while at the same time also having to triage other incoming emergency 911 calls for service.

- Multiple targeted GCIs were scheduled as soon as possible for homogenous groups affected by the incident.

- Other FRC Team efforts were directed at proactively identifying those individuals not initially identified as needing support who showed delayed reactions or were dealing with multiple co-occurring stressors.

- This incident underscored how an "officer down" call has a uniquely disturbing and lingering impact on Tele-communicators who are "living and seeing" this incident in their mind's eye from start to finish, while at the same time also having to triage other incoming emergency 911 calls for service.

- The magnitude and far-reaching impact of this incident raised awareness, especially within the injured LEO's agency, of the value of the FRCP and its immediate on-scene response capabilities. It also led to later contract discussions with the affected agencies to ensure that resources could be in place to deliver competent crisis intervention services to their personnel in the event of future traumatic events.

Case Study #4: Child Fatality/Struck and Killed While Walking to School

Early morning at the start of the school year, an eleven-year-old female was hit by two separate vehicles, a school bus and privately owned vehicle. On-scene resuscitation efforts by EMS were unsuccessful, leaving many First Responders feeling powerless and helpless that they could not save the child's life.

Adding new challenges to the already horrific nature of this tragedy was its location, the community's main street, with close proximity to three schools, and the fact that many passersby witnessed the incident or its immediate aftermath.

Juvenile deaths are especially difficult for First Responders, particularly for those who are triggered because they also have children or grandchildren of the same or similar age. Calls of this nature involving the most vulnerable and at risk (e.g., children, someone with special needs, the elderly) are especially difficult to process. An additional triggering factor is that this tragedy occurred in a very common space where many residents and others would later observe a memorial marking the exact location of this child's untimely death.

The entire FRC Team deployed to the community, including going directly to the scene and helping the First Responders. The FRC Team also went to the child's school, just blocks away, to meet with administrative staff, teachers, volunteers, and the School Resource Officers (SRO). One of the SROs helped make the positive identification and procured the family's contact information so that the FRC Team could follow up with the bereaved family. The team then shifted to tend to the other First Responders, including firefighters at the nearby fire department that were first on scene. The FRC Team scheduled and facilitated a GCI the next day for all the impacted First Responders.

Juvenile deaths are especially hard for First Responders, particularly for those who also have children, and rank among the most difficult critical incidents to process.

Lessons Learned from Case #4

- Juvenile deaths are especially hard for First Responders, particularly for those who also have children, and rank among the most difficult critical incidents to process.

- The suddenness of the death and the violent, public manner in which it occurred exacerbated the difficulties for both First Responders and survivors-victims-witnesses.

- The sense of vulnerability concerning the safety and protection of children was heightened for all parents and school personnel who interpreted this child's death, like all others, as generationally wrong.

- Media attention gave appropriate validation to this incredible loss of a young child but it also triggered more anxiety for the First Responders by continuing to re-expose them to the tragedy.

- The time of day, location of the incident and high volume of traffic, both pedestrian and vehicle traffic, meant that there were multiple witnesses to this tragedy who were also traumatized at the beginning of what was supposed to be a normal school day.

- News of this tragedy elicited a community-wide wave of grief, particularly within the school system, and tested the school's resources and capacity to respond and cope effectively in a timely fashion, with such tragedies.

- The GCIs (which are valued at a higher dollar value than simple crisis calls), led by the FRC Team in the aftermath of this incident, exposes the toll of cumulative trauma and the collage of emotions ranging from powerlessness, anger, numbness, etc. The GCIs also revealed both the construc-

Case Study #4: Child Fatality

Case Study #4: Child Fatality	Type of Contact or Incident	# Contacts	Hours Committed by FRCP Team	Initiating Dept.	Other Agencies Involved	Acuity Level of Service for Chaplain	Estimated $ Value, Based on Hours
Day of Event	Crisis Call	30	8	FCSO	School System, SROs Teachers Bus Drivers	Very High	8 hours @ $125 per hour = $1000
Weeks after Event	Support	30	8	FCSO Communications	—	Very High	8 hours @ $125 per hour = $1000
Weeks after Event	GCIs	1	2	EMS/Fire		Very High	2 hours @ $200 per hour with 2 FRCP members = $800
One Year after Event	Follow-up Calls	6	3			Low	x hours @ $125 per hour = $375
TOTAL	4	67	21	3	3	Median = Very High	$3175

tive and destructive coping habits of First responders and, therefore, underscored the need for teaching wellness and resiliency to ALL First Responders to help them emotionally survive and learn from similar calls that will invariably come during the course of their careers.

- This incident also demonstrates how multiple triggers can be associated with only one incident—date, time of day, the physical siting of any yellow school bus, the sound of screeching tires, etc.—while dredging up a trove of other painful memories and images from previous difficult calls.

- For First Responders, added triggers can include not only those dredged up from past incidents but also ones they might anticipate on the next call involving a pediatric injury or death.

- Note that this tragedy like so many others happened in the midst of COVID-19-related risks which were incredibly high for First Responders, who, as essential workers, have been *continuously* exposed during COVID-19 assuming grave risks many of the public were able to avoid due to going dormant with remote work options and flexible hours designed to keep them safe and less stressed.

Case Study #5: Domestic Violence (DV) Survivor with Two-year-old Child Needs Safe Housing on a Holiday Weekend

On a Good Friday, the FRC Team's on-call chaplain received a call from the FCSO that a domestic violence survivor and her two-year-old child were in desperate need of housing. The FCSO Victim Services Coordinator normally tasked with such needs was off duty at the time. The chaplain immediately discovered that this situation was further complicated by the fact that the young mother might be COVID-19 positive. The chaplain found that with this call and previous calls of this nature that few shelters answer phones in the late afternoon, with direct help being even harder to find after work hours. When the chaplain finally estab-

Note that this tragedy like so many others happened in the midst of COVID-19-related risks which were incredibly high for First Responders, who, as essential workers, have been continuously exposed during COVID-19 assuming grave risks many of the public were able to avoid...

lished contact with one shelter, he was told the mother would need COVID-19 testing prior to being granted shelter.

The FRC Team worked persistently for three hours with various shelters, our Coordinator for FaithHealth Community Engagement and others until a placement could be found at a battered women's shelter, pending a COVID-19 test at the AHWFB Emergency Department (ED) the next morning. The chaplain was able to collaborate with a FCSO Deputy to transport the mother to the ED for a rapid COVID-19 test, which enabled her to stay at the shelter.

Lessons Learned from Case #5

- This case demonstrates the persistence of the FRC Team in going above and beyond to address an emergent need and advocate for the most vulnerable at such a critical time for a mother and child.

- It also reveals the challenges of working within a system that is to often inefficient and far less proactive, even during normal work hours, and often inaccessible after hours and on holidays when the FRC Team and First Responders encounter some of the most vulnerable individuals and families that need *immediate* attention.

Case Study #5: Domestic Violence Survivor and Child Need Housing

Case Study #5: Housing Need	Type of Contact or Incident	# Contacts	Hours Committed by FRCP Team	Initiating Dept.	Other Agencies Involved	Acuity Level of Service for Chaplain	Estimated $ Value, Based on Hours
Day of Event	Resource Call	4	3	FCSO	Shelters; Hospital for COVID-19 testing	Low	3 hours @ $125 per hour = $375
Day after Event	Follow up with Agencies	2	2		Shelter		.2 hours @ $125 per hour = $25
TOTAL	2	6	5	1	3	Median = Low	$400

- The time and energy investment of over three hours by the FRC Team to ensure the safety of this mother and child is not atypical.

- This case and others like it should compel all community agencies to reexamine their capacity to address such emergencies during and after normal work hours/holidays, including having adequate backup systems, immediate access to emergency funds for essentials such as food and housing and efficient communications, NOT voicemail messages when a family is in crisis. It should never take three hours, under any circumstances, to resolve a crisis of this nature.

- What would have likely happened if the FRC Team did not answer this call for assistance?

Case Study #6: Responding to a Law Enforcement Retiree's Death (non-Line of Duty Death)

First Responder retirees collectively are part of the growing extended family of First Responders that includes both the retirees and those still actively serving. Because of these family connections, each retiree's death impacts the larger extended family of which he/she was a member. As is typical with many retiree deaths, the FRC Team already knew this retiree and had a shared history with the individual and his family. The on-call chaplain, immediately upon learning of the death from another retiree and verifying the death, reached out to the decedent's next of kin to offer the FRC Team's condolences and provide grief counselling and other ongoing support as needed.

However, a secondary but important role of the chaplain, was to ensure that the retiree's service would be appropriately recognized and honored by the agency he served in accordance with the retiree's and his family's wishes. This involved a series of logistical tasks for the chaplain, always working on behalf of the decedent's family. While each case presents unique challenges, these tasks always involve immediately sending a notification of the retiree's death to the Command Staff of the impacted agency,

First Responder retirees collectively are part of the growing extended family of First Responders that includes both the retirees and those still actively serving.

followed by an agency-wide notification that includes the retiree community and confirming an accurate work history for the decedent by conferring with Human Resources. In this case, once arrangements and work history were verified, the information was posted with the family's permission on the Hospital-Carelist (HCL) to be disseminated agency-wide.

In accordance with the retiree's wishes, the FRC Team made certain that all appropriate honors that can be bestowed on the retiree and his/her family were offered, including activation/use of the agency's Honor Guard, assistance with finding pallbearers (if burial is traditional), scheduling patrol escorts for processionals, establishing direct links using cell numbers between funeral home directors and the appropriate agency personnel as well as the FRC Team to ensure the as near perfect coordination as possible of all roles/tasks associated with the visitation/funeral. Family requests for the FRC Team's assistance in planning or officiating the funeral are not unusual.

A line of duty death (LODD) of an actively serving LEO, as will be described in Case Study #19, is immensely more complicated in multiple ways.

Lessons Learned from Case #6

- Each of these connections always generates a cascade of phone calls, emails and texts that are very time sensitive and can take hours to complete. It's critical to note that there is *no* room for error as one misstep or dropped communication can have dire consequences for the family and the impacted agency.

- Beyond the funeral, the FRC Team pivots back to ongoing support for the bereaved family and creates recurring calendar reminders of the retiree's death, rebuilds the Outlook contact information on this deceased First Responder to now focus on the surviving spouse and children.

- The FRC Team must also ensure the agency's retiree database and the team's retiree distribution list reflects the retiree's death, whose name is now moved to a "deceased retirees list."

Case Study #6: Responding to Retiree Death

Case Study #6: Responding to Retiree Death	Type of Contact or Incident	# Contacts	Hours Committed by FRCP Team	Initiating Dept.	Other Agencies Involved	Acuity Level of Service for Chaplain	Estimated $ Value, Based on Hours
Day of Event	Spousal Contact, Documentation	4	2	FCSO		Moderate	2 hours @ $125 per hour = $250
Weeks after Event	Support/Led Memorial Service	8	4	FCSO Communications		Moderate	8 hours @ $125 per hour = $1000
One Year after Event	Follow-up Calls	1	1			Low	1 hour @ $125 per hour = $125
TOTAL	5	13	7	2		Median = Moderate	$1375

- As is true with the public, all of these protocols for memorializing First Responder retirees have been made more challenging by COVID-19, which placed restrictions on how individual families and the affected agencies are allowed to grieve the deaths of so many of our public servants.

- It must be noted that the logistics surrounding a line of duty death (LODD) of an actively serving LEO is immensely more complicated compared to a First Responder retiree death. While some of the FRC Team's logistical tasks are similar to those involved in the natural or accidental death of a retiree, additional challenges and protocols immediately present in the case of a LODD. This is especially evident regarding its traumatic impact on the involved agency (institutional grief) and the community at large due to extensive media coverage. Understandably, the funeral is also more complicated and for this reason

After receiving a walking "debrief" from one of the on-scene supervisors as to what he believed had occurred (an overdose death with subject found first by peers, then parents), the chaplain made his way through the crowded home to locate the parents, both of whom had retreated to separate locations.

almost every First Responder agency has LODD protocols clearly stipulated in agency policies to ensure that appropriate honors are meticulously observed, including all notifications, the wearing of mourning bands and the mourning period for the entire agency, to name just a few.

- LODDs of LEOs also receive national attention and recognition on the Officer Down Memorial Page[7] once the impacted agency provides supporting documentation. Additionally, the agency must assist the decedent's family with the important but arduous process regarding local, state and federal death benefits. Note that similar websites, such as the National Fallen Firefighters Association, document and archive the LODDs of other First Responders in addition to providing many other resources to firefighters and their families.

Case Study #7: Overdose Death of Adolescent (pre-COVID-19)

The FRC Team was notified via CAD message very early on a weekend morning that an adolescent had been found deceased at home where he lived with his parents and siblings. Upon arrival the on-call chaplain found a houseful of family members and peers of the decedent, many of whom were grieving intensely. After receiving a walking "debrief" from one of the on-scene supervisors as to what he believed had occurred (an overdose death with subject found first by peers, then parents), the chaplain made his way through the crowded home to locate the parents, both of whom had retreated to separate locations. The next 2.5 hours for the chaplain were spent moving between multiple rooms of the house and backyard, all in an attempt to console the parents, other relatives who had arrived in waves and approximately eight peers of the decedent who had congregated away from the immediate family members.

Additionally, the chaplain was monitoring four groups of First Responders who were present. These included the firefighters who arrived just after the medics who were now leaving after establishing confirmation of death, the patrol officers who had arrived first and were now protecting the crime scene and the investigators who arrived last and would remain present as long as the investigation required and until the body transport to the morgue could be arranged. The chaplain, with the permission of parents, notified the impacted school personnel, conferred with the SRO assigned to that school, spoke with other relatives and the adolescent's employer. As is typical in most cases, the chaplain was the last responder to leave the residence after the family was allowed some moments of silence with the adolescent's covered body before it was transported and follow-up plans for ongoing support were established.

Lessons Learned from Case #7

- This case revealed the expected and overwhelming grief with the full gamut of reactions (sadness, anger, blaming, guilt, projection onto others, etc.) that accompanies the sudden, preventable and what is perceived to be the senseless death of a young person. For the parents this was especially devastating but also very impactful for the siblings, peers and grandparents (who experienced double grief over the loss of a grandchild combined with sharing the pain the death inflicted on their own adult children).

- For the First Responders on scene, this was an all too familiar tragedy, as many of them, prior to this call, had long since grown tired of administering NARCAN (naloxone HCL), sometimes repeatedly to save the same individuals, and only later struggle to process these losses as they go from one call to the next. Those First Responders with children of a similar age who had a front row seat at this tragedy hurt more deeply.

- The overall impact of this death was magnified by high levels of sensory exposure for those who discovered the body (parents/siblings/peers) but also for the on-scene First Responders who had the closest proximity for an extended time with the child (administering NARCAN,

This case revealed the expected and overwhelming grief with the full gamut of reactions (sadness, anger, blaming, guilt, projection onto others, etc.) that accompanies the sudden, preventable and what is perceived to be the senseless death of a young person.

moving/touching/examining the body, all while being surrounded by personal artifacts in the adolescent's room and elsewhere in the home).

- Such a death can and often does result in some stigma being felt by parents, the affected neighbors, the adolescent's teachers, school administrative staff, peer group, etc.

- For both parents and First Responders there is often shared anger focused on those individuals who are profiting from the distribution of drugs with no regard to the human costs. It's not uncommon in such cases for parents/other family members to want to launch their own "investigation" into who provided the drugs and "killed" their child.

Case Study #7: Overdose of an Adolescent

Case Study #7: Overdose of a Teenager	Type of Contact or Incident	# Contacts	Hours Committed by FRCP Team	Initiating Dept.	Other Agencies Involved	Acuity Level of Service for Chaplain	Estimated $ Value, Based on Hours
Day of Event	Crisis Call	12	4	FCSO	EMS	Very High	4 hours @ $125 per hour = $500
Day after Event	Support (Family)	4	3	—	School System	High	3 hours @ $125 per hour = $375
Weeks after Event	Support	4	2	—	—		2 hours @ $125 per hour = $250
One Year after Event	Follow-up Calls	2	1	–	—	Moderate	1 hour @ $125 per hour = $125
TOTAL	4	22	10	—	—	Median = Moderate	$1250

- Such a death reverberates through multiple communities, neighborhoods, the child's school, employer, the responding agencies, social media, etc.

- The death obviously had a unique impact on siblings and the peer group, who lack the coping resources to adequately care for themselves and each other. The peers in this case already knew multiple peers who had died in the previous year of a similar cause (overdose).

- This case shined a bright light on what still remains one of our greatest societal challenges...the extent of substance use, particularly opioids...and how overdose deaths impact all of us (faith communities, schools, hospitals, government agencies, drug treatment/rehab centers and others).

- The FRC Team made a recurring calendar reminder of this death to track this family in addition to providing some immediate follow-up for the parents and siblings, linking them to other resources. Saving the child's obituary with contact information for the parents is a part of the team's routine archiving and documenting these difficult calls.

Case Study #8: Salute to Fallen First Responders Across the Region When Their Bodies Are Escorted from the Medical Center

Since the inception of the FRCP, it has become customary for the FRC Team to be physically present whenever any First Responder's body is escorted from the medical center following a postmortem examination. This practice has been upheld for both LODD and non-LODD deaths on multiple occasions to honor the public service of the deceased First Responder and to offer the FRC Team's support to the many colleagues and family members who are present on AHWFB's Winston-Salem campus when this solemn transfer occurs.

The FRC Team's role traditionally includes receiving the First Responder's flag-draped body as it exits the morgue, accompanying the body, flanked by Honor Guard members from the fallen

Such a death reverberates through multiple communities, neighborhoods, the child's school, employer, the responding agencies, social media, etc.

First Responder's agency, from the morgue to a large outside gathering. Included are bereaved family members, more Honor Guard members, First Responders from multiple agencies and medical center Security Officers, with all uniformed personnel standing at attention and saluting as the First Responder's body comes into view. All non-uniformed attendees stand reverently with hands covering hearts. Many are sobbing with others choking back tears.

A very brief ceremony then ensues with a FRC Team member inviting family members and peers to encircle their loved one's flag-draped body. A prayer is then offered before the First Responder's body is transferred usually to a nearby hearse. The FRC Team then offers support to family and others present before the slow processional from the medical center begins.

The FRC Team is grateful for its collaboration with Security Officers on campus who immediately notify the FRCP Director when the bodies of fallen First Responders have been received at the medical center. It should be noted that because LODDs receive extensive media coverage and are quickly broadcast throughout the state, the FRC Team is often already on alert and ready to mobilize. Protocols are then activated which involve not only the impacted First Responder agency but also multiple local agencies working together to ensure that one of their own colleagues is afforded the highest respect when his/her body leaves the medical center to be escorted home.

To cite just a few examples, in April 2021 the LODDs of two Watauga County, NC deputies brought hundreds of First Responders from that county but also from Forsyth and contiguous counties to stage near AHWFB to pay tribute and participate in the homebound processional for these two fallen deputies who were ambushed and fatally shot answering a call. In this case with two LODDs from one agency, the logistics were especially challenging. Dozens of family members arrived early in Winston-Salem at a reunification site prior to coming to the medical center to participate in the processional. The FRC Team was present at two different locations to offer support and prayers for the family. Emergency management, multiple law enforcement agencies, emergency services, Security Officers on campus and medical center personnel in the autopsy suite all united in this tightly coordinated demonstration of unity within the First Responder family. Hundreds of First Responder vehicles, many staging at Winston-Salem's local baseball stadium, joined in the processional as it departed the medical center. The same honor was shown by all the First Responder agencies in every county in route who joined the processional as it passed through their jurisdictions. Every bridge and overpass during the over 100-mile journey home was lined with parked First Responder vehicles with emergency lights strobing, and many displaying US Flags, with countless First Responders and citizens saluting the two fallen officers.

Every bridge and overpass during the over 100-mile journey home was lined with parked First Responder vehicles with emergency lights strobing, and many displaying US Flags, with countless First Responders and citizens saluting the two fallen officers.

Lessons Learned from Case #8:

- The far-reaching impact of LODDs is further illustrated in these rituals where First Responders from a wide-ranging area converge at the medical center in a time of grief to honor one of their own fallen comrades.

- Many smaller First Responder agencies must lean on larger agencies following a LODD. Because many have been fortunate to have never endured such a loss, they are ill-prepared to face the logistical and media challenges. Often, they have no established protocols for conducting LODD funerals or other resources, such as an Honor Guard Team or Public Information Officer (PIO). Smaller agencies can be especially burdened by staffing shortages and may have few if any Reserve Officer resources. However, there is usually an outpouring of interagency support to help work through these challenges so that even the smallest, most under-resourced agency receives the necessary help to aid its survival in the initial days following a LODD.

- Specifically, in the case of AHWFB, this ritual of transporting a fallen First Responder's body from the medical center is made more challenging by the physical environment. For example, the exit point from the Gray Building (location of the medical center's autopsy suite) is an unsightly, crowded alley that is not only very difficult to find and navigate, but a very inappropriate setting for gathering family members and other agencies for such a solemn event. For obvious reasons the clinical, laboratory environment inside Gray Building is also a highly unsuitable location for the FRC Team to meet with bereaved families and peers who are on the campus following such tragedies. Hopefully, there can continue to be discussions about two specific concerns. One is how to use AHWFB's Davis Chapel as a unification site for family members and the Honor Guard since it would offer a sacred location for the body to lie in state prior to the departure from AHWFB and provide more safety and comfort for the bereaved. A second concern is to explore another exit route out of the

Case Study #8: Salute to Fallen First Responders Across the Region When Their BodiesAre Escorted from the Medical CenterHonoring Fallen Comrades and Processional

Case Study #8: Honoring Comrades	Type of Contact or Incident	# Contacts	Hours Committed by FRCP Team	Initiating Dept.	Other Agencies Involved	Acuity Level of Service for Chaplain	Estimated $ Value, Based on Hours
Day of Event	Salute and Planning Processional	200	6	FCSO	EMS	Low to Moderate	6 hours @ $125 per hour = $750
Day of Event	Support for Family	20	1		—		1 hour @ $125 per hour = $125
Weeksafter Event	Follow-up Calls to Agency	2	1			Low	1 hour @ $125 per hour = $125
TOTAL	3	222	8			Median = Low to Moderate	$1,000

medical center that might be more efficient to avoid the congestion and inappropriate locations described above. This latter concern about how a First Responder's body should be moved into and out of the medical center also raises the question: Why do we/should we hide the deaths of our most valuable and vulnerable public servants from other hospital staff, visitors or the public?

- It's important to note that not every First Responder death is a LODD, whether the death occurs at the medical center while the First Responder is a patient or elsewhere while actively serving. However, every effort is made by the FRC Team to honor the bereaved families and impacted agencies in each case, regardless of cause of or location of the death whenever possible.

- It is also important to note that the transfer vehicle is not always a hearse. Depending on the First Responder's affiliation and other factors, it might be an ambulance or a fire apparatus.

Case Study #9: FRC Team's Care for the Law Enforcement Retiree Family

As stated elsewhere, a growing number of retirees comprise the extended First Responder family. While the FRC Team is highly responsive to their most acute crisis needs, providing home and hospital visitation, there are many other celebratory occasions and opportunities to show support and engage with this unique subgroup of First Responders. These include recognizing their birthdays and paying special recognition to other milestones, including their retirements. One of many examples is honoring the oldest living FCSO retirees and encouraging the entire FCSO Command Staff to congratulate them on their birtdays and other special anniversaries.

The FRC Team maintains an updated database containing the emergency contact information for every FCSO retiree and goes to great lengths to recognize the birthday of every retiree, as well

While the FRC Team is highly responsive to their most acute crisis needs, providing home and hospital visitation, there are many other celebratory occasions and opportunities to show support and engage with this unique subgroup of First Responders.

It's worth noting that many law enforcement agencies, including the FCSO, have strived to discover creative ways to support retirees during COVID-19 by scheduling drive by parades, surprising individual retirees at their homes with a physical show of support with scores of staff bearing gifts and showering attention on their veteran colleagues...

as all actively serving FCSO staff, so that no one's birthday is forgotten. In the case of the retirees, a birthday greeting, whether in the form of a phone call, text or email, is always appreciated and usually elicits more information from the retiree, such as a request for prayer for the retiree or a loved one about a range of issues, the announcement of a new grandchild...or it opens the door to a healing conversation with a retiree who could use a caring friend.

All the retirees, because they are considered part of the law enforcement "family" are always included on the FRC Team's HCL when appropriate so that others, including actively serving FCSO staff and their retired peers can stay apprised of who is dealing with illness, hospitalization or celebrating good news in their respective families.

Prior to COVID-19, the FRC Team routinely attended monthly in-person retiree breakfast gatherings. When these were suspended, the team scheduled Zoom meetings, as mentioned previously, to not lose touch with this vulnerable group. The FRC Team joins the FCSO in making every attempt to include the retirees in the life of the agency they served by inviting them to key events and holiday gatherings as well as other special meetings and community forums.

The FRCP Director has used the invaluable experiences he's gleaned from the retirees to teach the FRC Team about the history and resiliency of this group who collectively comprise the legacy of the FCSO.

It's worth noting that many law enforcement agencies, including the FCSO, have strived to discover creative ways to support retirees during COVID-19 by scheduling drive by parades, surprising individual retirees at their homes with a physical show of support with scores of staff bearing gifts and showering attention on their veteran colleagues, many of whom are chronically ill and homebound. The extended family members of retirees have also participated in these events which are captured with photos and video for both the agency and each retiree's family.

Lessons Learned from Case #9

- Every First Responder agency, not just law enforcement, would be well-served by caring for and honoring its retirees. This is a group that often feels an abrupt disconnection from a profession that radically changed their lives and the lives of their families, leaving them in many cases to suffer alone like wounded, damaged military veterans, poorly prepared for assimilation back into civilian life. While many are scripted to count down the days to their retirement, they often find that when their separation day arrives, they are shocked by how hard it is to leave behind the uniform and gear, the persona and hypervigilance that defined them for decades. Many report experiencing an identity crisis (as do some First Responder spouses) and feel forgotten. Others lament never having had a meaningful exit interview that would have shown respect for their service, but just as importantly, would have validated them personally and helped the agency benefit from their many years of invaluable service and experience.

- Many of the retirees, while they may have left their law enforcement or other First Responder career behind, are still relatively young and are an untapped resource at such a critical time when their mature wisdom accrued from long years of experience could be most useful. Some go on to find other meaningful jobs. Still others are eager to serve as volunteers, part-time staff or take initiative on their own to help mentor younger First Responders who could immensely benefit from the wisdom of a wise, seasoned retiree.

- The retirees are also not a monolithic group. Not only is there a broad age range considering that some retire in their 50s. They also are diverse in terms of interests, politics, hobbies, comfort level with technology, etc. The oldest retirees predated computers and email and are understandably amazed at the tools and technology (body cameras, Tasers, smartphones, keyless cars, car-mounted computers, real-time crime surveillance, drones, etc.) that

While many are scripted to count down the days to their retirement, they often find that when their separation day arrives, they are shocked by how hard it is to leave behind the uniform and gear, the persona and hypervigilance that defined them for decades.

are constantly being developed, updated and made available to their younger counterparts today.

- Most importantly, the retirees are the living memorials of the agencies they served. Because First Responder agencies are so reactive, they are not always diligent or skilled at preserving their own rich histories. So, as retirees age, many of them are much more cognizant than their younger counterparts of the critical need to capture and archive their experiences and memories for the benefit of the agency and the community. This history really serves as the backbone of each First Responder agency. So, it is imperative that young recruits in rookie classes and new hires in each agency have this history impressed upon them if they are to understand the importance of institutional loyalty and pride. Otherwise, they will lack the historical context for understanding their vital work and a sacred appreciation for those public servants who came before them, especially those who were injured or killed in the LOD.

Case Study #9: FRC Team's Care for the Law Enforcement Retiree Family

Case Study #9: Care for the Law Enforcement Retiree Family	Type of Contact or Incident	# Contacts	Hours Committed by FRCP Team	Initiating Dept.	Other Agencies Involved	Acuity Level of Service for Chaplain	Estimated $ Value, Based on Hours
Monthly	Retiree Illnesses, Death, Calls, Meetings, Hospital Visits, E-mail Distributions, Texts	40	10	FCSO		Low	Minimum Average of 10 hours @ $125 per hour = $1250
TOTAL	8	40	10			Median = Low	$1250, but priceless

Case Study #10: FRC Team's Care for the Forsyth County Law Enforcement Detention Center (FCLEDC) Staff

The FRC Team regularly interacts with FCLEDC staff, which comprises both certified Detention Officers and civilian staff as well as contracted health providers. The team's services include both on-scene responses to critical incidents and many other services. Some examples of on-scene responses include the team's activation when:

- A staff member or a member of his/her family has a medical emergency requiring treatment or hospitalization.

- A staff member experiences a behavioral health crisis.

- A staff member suffers a high level of sensory exposure either from being assaulted by an inmate, responding to the serious injury, suicide attempt or death of an inmate by suicide or any other cause, exposure to a biohazard, etc.

- A staff member accompanies an inmate to the medical center after a serious medical emergency that, depending on outcome, has the potential to impact multiple groups of individuals including FCLEDC staff, on-site contract health providers, the inmate and his/her family, hospital staff and others.

The FRC Team, as it does with all of its other First Responder colleagues, also routinely spends time with Detention officers and other staff in less acute settings by attending muster (shift change) meetings, Command Staff meetings and other events. All of these non-critical meetings help accrue the trust so vital when a crisis erupts and the FRC Team needs immediate access to such a highly secure setting as the LEDC.

Some of the FRC Team's effectiveness is well demonstrated in a few examples. One involved rendering support to an armed Detention Officer (ADO) on AHWFB's Winston-Salem campus. ADO's routinely must accompany all inmates who are transported from LEDC to the medical center for treatment. In this case, an altercation between the ADO and the inmate in the ADO's custody resulted in the ADO suffering a medical emergency while in the ED. The FRC Team member on-call was able to respond immediately after being notified by the ADO's Chain of Command (COC) to offer support, assist in notifying family members and later provide care during this ADO's rehabilitation which ended with a very successful recovery.

A second example involved multiple FRC Team members deploying to the LEDC when on-duty staff received the tragic news that one of their own, a fellow Detention Officer, had died of complications from a chronic illness. This staff member's team, hearing of this death during their work shift, was grief-stricken and needed immediate on-scene support. The FRC Team spent hours on site and followed up with the deceased Detention Officer's peer group as well as assisted with supporting the Detention Officer's family in helping with the logistics and observance of protocols necessitated by the occurrence of an active employee's death.

A third example involves the FRC Team's multiple activations to attend to LEDC staff needs when groups of Detention Officers while working the same shift have been involved in rescue efforts when an inmate has attempted or completed suicide.

Lessons Learned from Case #10

- Detention Officers (more generally referred to as Correctional Officers around the nation) comprise a unique subset of First Responders within law enforcement agencies. As such, they have a strong affinity with one another to counteract the multiple stressors of their work.

- This cohesiveness is driven by an understandable mistrust of others and can aid their resilience. However, as with many other First Responder groups, it also has an incestuous component and can displace the important role one's immediate family should have. It can also lead to isolation, but it can unite them especially when one of them is injured or when their team members are confronted with grief.

- Detention Officers are often immersed in the negativity of other individuals' lives since they are charged with safeguarding and protecting those who, for one reason or another, have ended up incarcerated. Other First Responders, in contrast, generally have more opportunities to connect with more positive experiences during the course of their workdays. Detention Officers, on the other hand, are confined along with those they are committed to protecting. Self-care for them involves stomaching this aspect of the work, which even other First Responders would find intolerable, without letting its cumulative toll contaminate and impair their personal lives.

- Compounding these stressors is the fact that their work is mostly invisible to the public whose only understanding of the stressors and unique aspects of a Detention Officer's day-to-day work experiences are derived primarily from television. These false perceptions and lack of knowledge often result in a severe lack of validation for Detention Officers and, by association, their families, compared to other First Responders associated with law enforcement agencies whose work is more visible to and better understood and validated by the public.

- This lack of validation is unfortunate and ignores the unique challenges Detention Officers face. Though they are selected and trained to work in such a unique environment, classroom instruction alone cannot possibly prepare them to deal with all of the trauma and sensory exposure they will experience over the course of their careers.

- While all First Responders are and have always been essential frontline workers, COVID-19 poses even greater dangers for all the First Responders working in detention environments across the nation since these are congregant settings and therefore present many public health risks. The chronic stress of COVID-19 continues to weigh heavy on all personnel who work in such settings and also generates much anxiety for their family members, as well as for all those incarcerated and their families.

While all First Responders are and have always been essential frontline workers, COVID-19 poses even greater dangers for all the First Responders working in detention environments across the nation since these are congregant settings and therefore present many public health risks.

- Due to the LEDC, like all correctional facilities, having to be such a highly secure environment, the FRC Team's role responding within this environment requires extra training and compliance with strict protocols to help ensure the safety of all persons at the LEDC.

- Note that the Forsyth Jail and Prison Ministries (FJPM) is a non-profit ministry with a long history of serving inmates incarcerated in Forsyth County and their family members. However, this ministry is primarily site-based and limited to offering various programs for inmates at LEDC and a smaller, less secure prison in the County. In contrast, the FRCP is hospital-based and community-focused, connected to the all First Responder agencies and therefore capable of responding to traumatic events throughout the County and sometimes outside the County to deliver death notifi-

Case Study #10: Detention Center Injury and Follow Up

Case Study #10: Detention Center Injury and FollowUp	Type of Contact or Incident	# Contacts	Hours Committed by FRCP Team	Initiating Dept.	Other Agencies Involved	Acuity Level of Service for Chaplain	Estimated $ Value, Based on Hours
Day of Event	Crisis Calls	6	13	FCSO, Detention Center	Empowerment Homeless Program	Moderate	13 hours @ $125 per hour = $1625
Day after Event	Support- Attempted Family Notification	3	3				3 hours @ $125 per hour = $375
Weeks after Event	Support, Funeral	9	6				6 hours @ $125 per hour = $750
TOTAL	4	18	22	2	1	Median = Moderate	$2750

cations and other traumatic messages to inmates' family members. An example of a point of intersection for the FRCP and FJPM teams would be a critical incident that occurs at LEDC such as the suicide of an inmate. However, the FRC Team has the capability to not only deploy immediately to the LEDC to address a crisis impacting staff members, but can also deploy throughout the community to notify and support family members who are impacted by that and any other critical incident.

Case Study #11: Juvenile Homicide/Multi-agency Involvement

An early morning call from EMS requested the FRC Team's assistance following the death of a five year old. The team soon learned that the investigating law enforcement agency determined this death to be a homicide. The manner of death and prior abuse of the child intensified the impact of this incident for all First Responders on scene. Other circumstances, including the fact that the child was adopted and that the adoptive family was at the center of a homicide investigation also heavily impacted social workers as well as others in the adoptive care system who had a unique relationship to this child along with the foster family. The FRC Team provided direct in-person care in the form of a GCI to this latter group but also had multiple contacts with the involved First Responders. Approximately three months after this homicide, the FRC Team received a request from the care providers, all of whom were still grieving this loss, to plan and lead a memorial service to further aid them in their healing after such a senseless, traumatic death of a child.

Lessons learned from Case #11

- All cases involving the most vulnerable victim populations weigh heavily on First Responders and all of the involved care providers. This is especially true with the death of a young child as illustrated in this case and previous ones.

- Primary emotions after learning of the homicide of a child are anger, blame and overwhelming grief but also, for some at least, feelings of guilt as everyone searches for how the tragedy might have been prevented.

- Any death of a child feels generationally wrong with the intentional taking of the life of a child (homicide) being unconscionable.

- All those touched by this juvenile's death who were also parents found the impact of this case lingering much longer than the pain of other critical incidents, making it much more difficult to process.

- In addition to being highly ranked as a most difficult critical incident for First Responders, a child homicide, when added to other cumulative trauma in the careers of First Responders, can be disabling and even career-ending.

Case Study #11: Juvenile Homicide with Multi-agency Involvement

Case Study #11: Juvenile Homicide with Multi-agency Involvement	Type of Contact or Incident	# Contacts	Hours Committed by FRCP Team	Initiating Dept.	Other Agencies Involved	Acuity Level of Service for Chaplain	Estimated $ Value, Based on Hours
Day of Event	Crisis Call	4	4	EMS	DSS	Very High	4 hours @ $125 per hour = $500
Months after Event	Support (memorial service planning)	4	4	EMS		Moderate	4 hours @ $125 per hour = $500
TOTAL	2	8	8	EMS		Median = High	$1000

- Involvement of the criminal justice system (CJS), although a necessary component of every criminal case, vastly complicates and delays the grieving process and provides many triggers that can often cause a resurgence of grief.

- The original requestor of help, EMS, and all of its staff have the FRC Team's contact information and knew that the team would immediately mobilize after being informed of this incident. EAP nor any other entity available has the capacity to be this responsive at all hours and go to the point of need.

- Calls involving the serious injury of a child, or, as in this case, the violent death of child are also impactful on the FRC Team and make self-care an imperative.

Calls involving the serious injury of a child, or, as in this case, the violent death of child are also impactful on the FRC Team and make self-care an imperative.

Case Study #12: Threat to Public Health Staff While Conducting Site Inspection

Two Public Health (PH) supervisors contacted the Program Director late one afternoon requesting the FRC Team's support for two of their employees who had just been threatened while conducting a routine site inspection at a local business. The business owner, who had a history of being difficult in previous encounters with PH staff, became verbally aggressive and displayed a weapon. The two PH employees were able to quickly and safely exit this environment and report the incident to their supervisors who immediately sought assistance to help them cope with this traumatic incident. An FRC Team member immediately deployed to a safe location to meet with the two employees and their supervision to provide on-site in-person support and establish plans for follow up.

Lessons learned from Case #12

- As stated elsewhere, many of the staff serving in PH, Social Services and similar departments can be considered to be quasi-First Responders in that their community-based work carries clear safety risks that include transitioning to multiple locations and dealing with all kinds of clients in varying stages of need and distress.

- As this case indicates, local government employees, such as PH staff, can be the target of blame and rage from disgruntled citizens.

- A complicating factor is that the chronic stressors and socio-economic inequities across all communities have become even more difficult to manage and have been exacerbated by the intense polarization on many levels as a result of COVID-19.

- This case also reveals the high level of sensory exposure that can result from a site visit that quickly becomes volatile and threatening when a business owner displays a weapon in the presence of two defenseless PH workers simply doing their jobs.

- In addition, this case raises concerns about the risk of a recurrence, not only for these staff members but for all PH employees who have similar roles that might subject them to similar grave risks.

Case Study #12: Threat to Public Health Staff While Conducting Site Inspection

Case Study #12: Threat After Inspection	Type of Contact or Incident	# Contacts	Hours Committed by FRCP Team	Initiating Dept.	Other Agencies Involved	Acuity Level of Service for Chaplain	Estimated $ Value, Based on Hours
Day of Event	Crisis Call	4	3	Public Health	FSCO	High	3 hours @ $125 per hour = $375
Day after Event	Support	3	1			Moderate	1 hour @ $125 per hour = $125
TOTAL	2	7	4		1	Median = High	$500

- The increasing prevalence of guns has understandably elevated all of these risks for our community's unarmed public servants who interact daily with some individuals who can become hostile and have easy access to weapons.

- The case also provides a strong rationale for adding a new dimension to the in-service training for many of our unarmed public servants to help them deal with a range of traumatic incidents that can potentially impair their functioning both at work and at home.

Case Study #13: Homicide of a Local College Student and Its Impact on Multiple Families/Communities

A command level law enforcement supervisor contacted the Program Director about the homicide of a local college student in an adjacent county, explaining that she had been murdered by her estranged boyfriend. Furthermore, the supervisor stated that the decedent's best friend at the same campus was a daughter of a law enforcement colleague known by the supervisor and the Program Director. An FRC Team member was immediately connected to the parents of the bereaved daughter to offer multiple levels of support and referrals to each of them, including an in-person meeting with the daughter.

Lessons Learned from Case #13

- This case demonstrates the deep ties between law enforcement officers and their loyalty to one another. As is often the case, First Responders are acutely aware when any critical incident, especially one involving death, impacts one of their own. This includes homicides and other crimes that happen regionally and are quickly shared through a tight interagency and peer network.

- The Program Director has a longstanding relationship with the referring supervisor and the law enforcement father of the bereaved student whose best friend had been

The increasing prevalence of guns has understandably elevated all of these risks for our community's unarmed public servants who interact daily with some individuals who can become hostile and have easy access to weapons.

brutally murdered. This networking expedited getting help to both the parents and daughter within hours of learning of the tragedy.

- This death also underscored how difficult it is for First Responders to deal with their own grief and the traumas that impact their own families. By necessity they must compartmentalize much of the grief they see in their day-to-day work. However, incidents such as this homicide that impacted one of their own cause them to over-identify and feel powerless. They also struggle with how to support their own families when their work has often left them so emotionally calloused.

- First Responders also typically are very over-protective of their own children, regardless of their age. So, this case generated fear and anxiety for all law enforcement families who knew about this incident. The young age and innocence of the victim also made this horrible crime even more egregious.

- First Responders, because they are so familiar with the CJS, also know how criminal cases can immensely complicate the homicide survivor family's grief.

Case Study #13: Homicide of a Local College Student and Its Impact on Multiple Families/Communities

Case Study #13: College Student Murder	Type of Contact or Incident	# Contacts	Hours Committed by FRCP Team	Initiating Dept.	Other Agencies Involved	Acuity Level of Service for Chaplain	Estimated $ Value, Based on Hours
Day of Event	Crisis Call	4	2	FCSO	EMS	Very High	2 hours @ $125 per hour = $250
Weeks after Event	Support	2	2		—	Moderate	2 hours @ $125 per hour = $250
TOTAL	2	6	4			Median = High	$500

Case Study #14: Multiple-Fatality Fire Call

A Fire Captain contacted the Program Director on behalf of his peers requesting assistance to lead a GCI for approximately 30 firefighters who had been involved in responding to a multi-fatality fire call the previous night. Among the three decedents was an infant with one of the adult victims dying later at the hospital. An FRC Team member was able to help facilitate this GCI with the assistance of some peer team members.

Lessons learned from Case #14

- This case met all the criteria for being classified and treated as a critical incident based on universal CISM (Critical Incident Stress Management) practices.

- This was true with respect to the magnitude of the fire itself but also the loss of life. Three on-scene resuscitation attempts (CPR) with three different victims were unsuccessful, resulting in three fatalities, one of whom was an infant.

- The heaviness of this incident in terms of loss of life and other challenges of getting all emergency personnel to what was a chaotic scene made this a tough call for even the veteran firefighters.

- The level of sensory exposure had a major impact as well, especially on all firefighters with children of their own. For some of the youngest firefighters this was their first infant/child death and first experience performing or witnessing CPR on an infant/child at a scene with multiple victims in one dwelling.

- While emergency services (Fire and EMS) are the primary responders on such calls, all First Responders, including law enforcement also present on scene, carry the memories of these calls not only when they leave their shifts but throughout their careers. After these types of calls, reconnections with their own families and especially their children are powerful reminders of the impact and risks inherent in their work. As they observe their own children in

While emergency services (Fire and EMS) are the primary responders on such calls, all First Responders, including law enforcement also present on scene, carry the memories of these calls not only when they leave their shifts but throughout their careers.

healthy and safe environments, they are filled with gratitude but always mindful of the pain and grief accompanying their work.

- Firefighters also expend a lot of energy and time in educating the public about fire safety to avert such tragedies from ever happening. Therefore, it is very difficult to reconcile why all businesses and homes would not regularly use and maintain smoke detectors. Firefighters are justifiably angry after these tragedies whenever they discover that, in many cases, one working nine-volt battery could have saved lives.

- The firefighter culture is often better equipped for constructive coping in the aftermath of such calls and is, therefore, more resilient than other First Responder groups due to periods of sustained contact with one another while working long shifts. The experience of congregant life in fire stations, while continuously training, maintaining equipment and sharing daily activities like eating meals together, all combine to build trust and create a strong and

Case Study #14: Multiple-Fatality Fire Call

Case Study #15: Multiple-Fatality and Fire Call	Type of Contact or Incident	# Contacts	Hours Committed by FRCP Team	Initiating Dept.	Other Agencies Involved	Acuity Level of Service for Chaplain	Estimated $ Value, Based on Hours
Day of Event	Crisis Call and GCI	30	4	EMS		Very High	4 hours @ $200 per hour with 2 staff = $800
Weeks after Event	Support	2	4			Moderate	4 hours @ $125 per hour = $500
TOTAL	3	32	8			Median = High	$1300

enduring sense of family within the fire service. This affinity also bodes well for better quality of life in retirement for firefighters. The tradition of multiple family members growing up in and joining the fire service also strengthens these bonds and provides a source of tremendous pride.

- Firefighters are also less reluctant to reach out for help as a group because of this cohesiveness and belief in self-care. Additionally, firefighters on a national level have ascribed more strongly to the benefits of CISM than other First Responder groups. However, since some growing evidence questions the efficacy of CISM for First Responders, it may be that the shared belief firefighters have in one other, their passion for their work and sense of family, benefit them as much as the interventions themselves. High levels of accessibility to the FRC Team enhances these intrinsic strengths.

- One redemptive outcome of this tragedy is that it provided the FRC Team with an additional opportunity to build trust with these firefighters who, in addition to needing peer support after such difficult calls, also need highly responsive chaplaincy services to augment this internal support and address many existential and personal issues that are often dredged up after this level of sensory exposure.

Case Study #15: Assault on a Law Enforcement District Office, Presenting a High Threat to Public Safety and Linked to Intra-familial Homicides

The FRC Team received multiple notifications including direct phone calls to the Program Director and other alerts that a male subject had attacked a law enforcement district office with an assault weapon before fleeing and leading all local law enforcement agencies on a dangerous pursuit that culminated in one of the city's most popular parks on a busy afternoon. Miraculously, no First Responders or civilians were killed or injured in the initial attack or over the course of the protracted incident that tra-

One redemptive outcome of this tragedy is that it provided the FRC Team with an additional opportunity to build trust with these firefighters who, in addition to needing peer support after such difficult calls, also need highly responsive chaplaincy services to augment this internal support and address many existential and personal issues that are often dredged up after this level of sensory exposure.

The case easily
qualifies as a
major critical
incident due to
the massive,
multi-agency
response,
the chaos,
complexity and
expansiveness of
multiple crime
scenes, the
grave threat it
imposed on the
public as it
migrated from
the initial location
of the assault,
through several
densely-populated
streets and
neighborhoods
and its
culmination in a
public park...

versed the city. The perpetrator was eventually wounded, taken into custody, treated for his survivable injuries and charged with multiple crimes, including what would eventually be determined to be two homicides of his family members prior to the violent assault on law enforcement officers.

Lessons Learned from Case #15

- The case easily qualifies as a major critical incident due to the massive, multi-agency response, the chaos, complexity and expansiveness of multiple crime scenes, the grave threat it imposed on the public as it migrated from the initial location of the assault, through several densely-populated streets and neighborhoods and its culmination in a public park, adjacent to a high school, that was being used by scores of civilians of all ages who were enjoying an otherwise normal day of outdoor activities.

- While the pursuit itself put countless First Responders and the public at risk, the dangers at the park were numerous as arriving law enforcement officers had to find and isolate the suspect while also securing such a vast area filled with civilians, including adults and children.

- All of the civilians using the park along with other bystanders in the adjacent neighborhood, were shocked as they saw the park suddenly become surrounded within minutes by emergency vehicles and over a hundred law enforcement officers converging on the suspect's location.

- These same witnesses would later praise law enforcement officers for their bravery and efficient resolution to the crisis that kept the public safe and resulted in no casualties.

- The massive and rapid law enforcement response involving such a great expenditure of resources is even more notable considering concurrent challenges being faced by all law enforcement agencies, including staff shortages, a backlog of other investigations including homicide and other criminal investigations and overall fatigue during an extended period of coping with social unrest and increasing public scrutiny.

- Ongoing COVID-19 concerns, including a national lack of compliance across First Responder communities with vaccines, also created additional stressors for all First Responder agency heads who are struggling to balance public health concerns associated by COVID-19 with maintaining an adequate workforce to ensure public safety.

- Command level law enforcement staff are also concerned with how to balance the public's expectations for law enforcement protection while also safeguarding the well-being of individual officers and families who are facing multiple professional and personal stressors, including the cumulative stress of expanding workloads and difficult calls.

- The impact of sensory exposure was also notable for both young officers and even for seasoned investigators who have never experienced this kind of overload with pending death investigations.

- The media involvement in such an evolving and complex case is inevitable and important for informing the public. However, it can also bring added pressure to First Responders whose work is always under scrutiny. Fortunately, much-deserved public appreciation and validation of law enforcement's role was expressed in the aftermath of this incident.

- In terms of public impact, this incident was profound and extensive since all those affected could not be identified. Those in closest proximity to the scene at the time were clearly traumatized, but many others suffered vicarious trauma. A typical response from the public, in addition to being grateful for a peaceful resolution by law enforcement, was an intensely heightened sense of vulnerability... an acute awareness that if this can happen in a public park on a summer afternoon, then it can happen anywhere.

The media involvement in such an evolving and complex case is inevitable and important for informing the public. However, it can also bring added pressure to First Responders whose work is always under scrutiny.

Accompanying this sense of vulnerability was an understandable need to practice more vigilance in order to feel safe and resume normal activities.

- Fear of a recurrence was also a common response as concerns for personal safety and family members became more prominent. Other reactions included anger and confusion that one person's violent actions could be so disruptive to the quality of life of so many innocent witnesses who were enjoying their daily lives in what was perceived to be a safe location.

- This evolving community crisis tested the adaptability and responsiveness of the FRC Team to immediately deploy simultaneously to multiple locations, including the park itself, the impacted agency's public safety center to check on individual law enforcement officers and Tele-communicators, and then transition quickly to assist with death notifications once the two homicides were discovered and the incident rapidly became highly complex.

Case Study #15: Assault on a Law Enforcement District Office, Presenting a High Threat to Public Safety and Linked to Intra-familial Homicides

Case Study #15: Assault on Officer	Type of Contact or Incident	# Contacts	Hours Committed by FRCP Team	Initiating Dept.	Other Agencies Involved	Acuity Level of Service for Chaplain	Estimated $ Value, Based on Hours
Day of Event	Crisis Call	12	9	FCSO	EMS, Clemmons PD	Very High	9 hours @ $125 per hour = $1125
Weeks after Event	Support ; Follow-up Calls; 1:1 Conversations	8	4				4 hours @ $125 per hour = $500
TOTAL	4	20	13		2	Median = Very High	$1625

- In the midst of such a protracted and complicated incident and the ongoing transfer of vital information, the risk of doing irreparable harm is ever present and must be avoided at all costs. This is especially critical regarding the delivery of traumatic messages since there is no margin for error. The FRC Team's interactions with the First Responders, bereaved family members and all other individuals impacted by this crisis must always be highly competent and professional. This includes the FRC Team's meticulous care and advocacy at such a vulnerable time for the bereaved family members, attending to every possible need, but also working alongside family clergy representatives when they are present after such a horrific incident.

- The FRC Team's immediate on-scene assistance within minutes of being deployed was predicated on intricate, well-established webs of trust with all the involved agencies. The team also put multiple follow-up plans in place with various groups and individuals impacted by the incident.

Case Study #16: Unique Challenges and Considerations Viewing the Body After an Overdose Death

The FRC Team's on-call chaplain was activated by a Telecommunicator after a CAD (computer assisted dispatch) message alert of an overdose death was sent to the entire team. Upon arrival at the residence, a low-income apartment complex, the First Responder chaplain found the scene to be unusually chaotic and volatile. The responding law enforcement officers, though accustomed to dealing with similar unstable situations, were having to spend extra time and resources to protect themselves, other family members and the integrity of the crime scene. Since overdose deaths are treated as homicides until proven otherwise, a thorough investigation was required to determine the exact cause of death. A highly dysfunctional

The FRC Team's immediate on-scene assistance within minutes of being deployed was predicated on intricate, well-established webs of trust with all the involved agencies.

This incident strongly underscores the need for continuous pre-incident education and in-service training for all law enforcement officers over their career spans about the unique role of chaplains on scene at crisis calls...

family giving conflicting accounts and assigning blame to one another for what had transpired made everyone's role, including the First Responder chaplain's role, more difficult. The actions of some family members, including one family member who abruptly fled the scene, and the family's lack of cooperation with law enforcement investigators also generated distrust and communication challenges for all the First Responders who were trying to conduct a thorough investigation while keeping the scene safe. A history of violence and law enforcement's frequent calls to the area also justifiably increased the anxiety for First Responders on scene, as well the Telecommunicators, who were constantly monitoring this call.

As is typical on many crisis calls involving a death, the chaplain advocated for the family's right, if they so desire in each case, to have some quality time for a brief prayer and reflection with or in close proximity to their loved one's body whenever feasible and safe just prior to the decedent's body being transported to the medical center morgue. The chaplain, considering the unique circumstances of this death and the environment, carefully devised and shared a plan with the law enforcement officers in charge of the scene that would allow this important and healing ritual to occur. However, the situation devolved significantly when a single family member failed to comply and violated established boundaries as this ritual was taking place. This action robbed other family members of some healing closure and caused law enforcement officers to quickly intercede to establish control and expedite the transport of the body from the residence.

Lessons Learned from Case #16

- This incident strongly underscores the need for continuous pre-incident education and in-service training for all law enforcement officers over their career spans about the unique role of chaplains on scene at crisis calls and particularly the valuable role chaplains can have in attending to the needs of grief-stricken family members while also advocating for their law enforcement partners.

- This "being with" compassionate presence of chaplains with grieving families actually frees up law enforcement and crime scene investigators to do their critical investigative work unimpeded by distractions, including disruptive and uncooperative family members.

- A clearly understood delineation of everyone's roles prior to deploying to crises of this nature not only builds trust and understanding, but also allows for all First Responders to anticipate potential problems and challenges and better appreciate how a First Responder chaplain on scene can make their difficult jobs less stressful.

- This incident also offered a unique opportunity to explore the many misunderstandings still all too common among some First Responders, and especially law enforcement officers, regarding the family's right to view, except in very rare circumstances, or at least to be near their loved one's body for a brief period before it is transported from the scene where the death has occurred.

- "Viewing" in most cases is not, nor should it be (depending on cause of death and condition of the body), a full, uncovered viewing. Instead, viewing the body can be better understood in most cases as being allowed to have some degree of close proximity to the body even if a partial viewing or touching the decedent is not possible. It usually consists of family members, while being accompanied by the chaplain, being allowed to stand near a covered body, or, more precisely, the body bag containing the body, before it is transported.

- Research has shown and First Responder chaplains as well as bereaved family members can attest that families who are allowed this sacred time with their loved one's body, however brief or constrained the time might be by unusual circumstances, exhibit more constructive coping. Most importantly, this ritual conveys a deep sense of respect the FRC Team has for validating the family's loss and honoring

Most importantly, this ritual conveys a deep sense of respect the FRC Team has for validating the family's loss and honoring the decedent's life.

The chaplain's presence in this ritual serves as a reminder to all that no one's life should be judged solely by how it ends.

the decedent's life. The chaplain's presence in this ritual serves as a reminder to all that no one's life should be judged solely by how it ends.

- The FRC Team has found that this viewing ritual can elicit healthy grieving, not only for the bereaved family, but also for the First Responders who are present. The FRC Team invites into a circle of prayer around the gurney holding the decedent's body, whether the location is a hallway, front yard, garage or at the back door of an ambulance or other transport vehicle, as a powerful way of acknowledging the far-reaching repercussions each death has for everyone. At no time is this more evident that when another young person's life is senselessly lost due to a drug overdose, suicide or some other horrific accident that devastates not just families but often neighborhoods, schools and entire communities. First Responders see this devastation continuously and, as stated elsewhere, bear the cumulative impact of this life-altering sensory exposure over their careers. In turn, their family members are the victims of vicarious trauma as these tragic experiences invariably follow the First Responders home at the end of their shifts.

- Law enforcement officers, like all First Responders, are highly trained. However, unlike the FRC Team, they are not trained in understanding traumatic grief and caring for grief-stricken families who often are displaying a full range of emotions, some of which can be repulsive and easily misinterpreted as hostile or threatening by those who are untrained.

- Additionally, law enforcement officers are task-oriented, not process-oriented. This orientation and skill set serve law enforcement officers well and protects the public since they must be continuously vigilant and ready to react rapidly to protect life and property. However, this default reactive posture which requires a certain on-the-job compartmentalization of feelings that is appropriate in a para-military environment, can leave LEOs emotionally calloused, anxious and ill-prepared when they are not in their comfort zone of operating by procedures and checklists. Some LEOs, though not all, can be resistant to a family's right to view the decedent's body because *they* are anxious and trained to anticipate potential negative outcomes which can hinder them from seeing a positive healing outcome.

- If officers are to function effectively, some degree of objectification is also necessary since a critical need at every crime scene is the preservation of evidence and the chain of custody of that evidence. First Responders must also protect and treat the decedent's body as evidence along with many physical artifacts at a scene, something that can be extremely difficult for bereaved families and other witnesses to accept when they don't understand why a crime scene must be preserved and that an investigation can take hours and even days in some cases to be completed.

- Family members, on the other hand, are in a state of grief and shock as they struggle to assimilate their deeply personal loss. Consequently, they feel a desperate need to be near their loved one's body as a normal part of grieving and are comforted by being given the opportunity, contrary to what some First Responders fear might happen.

- Many bereaved families reflecting back on a loved one's death often report that they were experiencing a kind of tunnel vision that left them oblivious to the all the "strangers" or "uninvited guests" (First Responders, neighbors, others) who had suddenly been mobilized and converged on their home. What was previously a private living space can within minutes become an active "scene."

- The Program Director attests that after facilitating this viewing ritual for hundreds of families, it is always appreciated and, to the surprise of some law enforcement officers, it instantly creates a sacred bond and renewed understanding on the part of bereaved families and the officers who were with them at such a life-transforming

Many bereaved families reflecting back on a loved one's death often report that they were experiencing a kind of tunnel vision that left them oblivious to the all the "strangers" or "uninvited guests" (First Responders, neighbors, others) who had suddenly been mobilized and converged on their home.

time. Conversely, family members who feel straightjack-eted and forced to be isolated from their loved one's body at a scene long past the time when this is necessary, grow increasingly anxious and angry if they are callously told "You can see him/her at the funeral home."

- Many individuals and families who may have harbored ill will toward law enforcement over some previous alter-cations are immediately disarmed when they experience heartfelt compassion being displayed by LEOs and other First Responders who are not afraid to stand with them in their suffering, even if it is just to respect their home envi-ronment, offer sincere condolences or check back with them days later. Such kindnesses are expressed by many First Responders individually, but unfortunately often with-out the public's knowledge or appreciation.

- On behalf of all First Responders it must be noted that the public often forgets the personal and institutional grief being carried by all our public servants in addition to what

Case Study #16: Unique Considerations and Challenges–Family Viewing the Body After an Overdose Death

Case Study #17: Drug Overdose and Family Viewing	Type of Contact or Inci-dent	# Con-tacts	Hours Com-mitted by FRCP Team	Initiating Dept.	Other Agencies Involved	Acuity Level of Service for Chap-lain	Esti-mated $ Value, Based on Hours
Day of Event	Crisis Call	8	4	FCSO	Public Safety Center	High	4 hours @ $125 per hour = $500
Days after Event	Meeting, Calls	4	2	Public Safety Center		Moderate	2 hours @ $125 per hour = $250
TOTAL	3	12	6		1	Median = High	$750

they experience daily on difficult calls. The suffering they endure with sickness and death in their own personal families is made even heavier by those losses within their respective work families. This has been especially true as COVID-19 has, sadly, claimed more First Responders' lives in 2020-2021 than any other cause of death.[8]

- Taken together, all these challenges should help us understand why First Responders justifiably have a jaundiced worldview and are so deserving of our support and compassion as they are reminded daily of the fragility of life and compelled to confront their own mortality.

- Finally, this case illustrates why the FRC Team must always maintain poise and competence while in close proximity to the intense suffering and confusion being experienced by family members, many of whom have just received or learned of the worst news of their lifetimes.

Case Study #17: Motor Vehicle Accident (MVA) Fatality Impacting First Responders and Bystander Witnesses

Leaders from a local fire department reached out to the Program Director the day following a horrific single vehicle crash that instantly killed the operator. Initial descriptions about the nature of the call, the crash scene and condition of the victim flagged this as a major critical incident for all the First Responders on scene. A group crisis intervention (GCI), to be facilitated by two FRC Team members, was scheduled at the impacted department within hours of this request for help.

Lessons Learned from Case #17

- The FRC Team members immediately confirmed at the GCI that every First Responder on this call was deeply affected. That is not always the case where more seasoned firefighters can often console their younger counterparts. However, this call was distressing even to the veterans,

Taken together, all these challenges should help us understand why First Responders justifiably have a jaundiced worldview and are so deserving of our support and compassion as they are reminded daily of the fragility of life and compelled to confront their own mortality.

*First Responders
can typically
remember vivid
details of some
of their first calls
on the front end
of their careers,
especially the
graphic images
that often linger
with them for
decades even
into retirement.*

some of whom had decades of experience answering some of the worst calls involving fatalities. Three of these veterans rated this incident their worst or second worst of their entire careers, which collectively spanned over 100 years in the fire service.

- The high levels of sensory exposure account for the severe distress accompanying this call. Key elements included the violent manner of death (projection from the vehicle at a high rate of speed), the graphic, mutilated condition of the body and the accident debris field which amplified the exposure for all First Responders present and complicated management of the scene.

- This critical incident reveals the cumulative trauma experienced over decades, as it dredges up or resurrects past incidents. First Responders can typically remember vivid details of some of their first calls on the front end of their careers, especially the graphic images that often linger with them for decades even into retirement.

- As mentioned previously, it is important to understand and appreciate the extended family culture that thrives in those fire departments which rely heavily on volunteers who bravely sacrifice many hours of their personal time responding to horrific tragedies, attending training and giving back in countless and selfless ways to their communities.

- This affinity and cohesiveness aids in fostering resiliency and trust. However, because the fire service has always had a strong family tradition, adolescents as junior firefighters can inadvertently be exposed to trauma that can be incapacitating even for adults, as this call demonstrated. A universal challenge for fire departments is how to preserve and honor the noble tradition of introducing young family members into the fire service, while also making certain these most vulnerable and inexperienced First Responders are prepared for and protected from the physical and emotional hazards as much as possible, while also gaining experience.

- In this case the decedent was young, making this tragic death especially untimely and premature. The decedent was also known by some of the First Responders and was a distant relative of another. These relational ties serve as a reminder that First Responders serving in some more rural communities run the high risk daily of deploying to incidents to find that the victims are their neighbors, friends, fellow firefighters and even their own family members. Obviously, the potential trauma for the First Responders who are related to the victims can be intense.

- Every incident of this nature that happens on a public roadway or in a neighborhood also carries the additional risks that innocent bystanders, passersby or neighbors (adults and children) can be and often are abruptly exposed to scenes and images that can leave them stunned as if they have stumbled upon the carnage typical of a gruesome action movie. A civilian couple who happened to be driving by in the immediate aftermath of this tragedy reached out to the involved fire department the next day and were immediately directed to the FRC Team which provided in-person assistance to help this couple process their anomalous experience.

- The popularity of social media and the ubiquitous presence of smartphones also create serious concerns for First Responders and the FRC Team since any disaster or accident scene can easily be photographed, videoed and uploaded in minutes without regard to the devastating impact of these actions. This is especially true when the scene is highly public and visible. Even if this use of media from a public right of way in the midst of a tragedy is legal, it is extremely offensive to First Responders and dishonors their work, as it also disrespects those killed or injured as well as their family members who, in many cases, have not yet been officially notified of their loved one's injury or death.

The popularity of social media and the ubiquitous presence of smartphones also create serious concerns for First Responders and the FRC Team since any disaster or accident scene can easily be photographed, videoed and uploaded in minutes without regard to the devastating impact of these actions.

- Typically, chaplaincy services for fire departments around the region and nation has for many decades been provided by local clergy who reside in the same communities. These trusted local clergy are invaluable and are to be commended for their volunteer service. However, much more can and should be done to forge valuable networks with these volunteer chaplains, the local fire departments they serve and the hospital-based chaplains who are anchored in community and regional medical centers.

- The FRC Team encourages the public to especially validate and honor the work of volunteer firefighters as they deal with daunting challenges made more difficult by COVID-19. The entire nation depends heavily on thousands of volunteer firefighters who greatly outnumber their paid counterparts in urban, municipal fire departments. According to the National Fire Protection Association (NFPA) there were an estimated 1,115,000 career and volunteer firefighters in the United States in 2018. Of the total number of firefighters 370,000 (33%) were career firefighters and 745,000 (67%) were volunteer firefighters.[9]

Case Study #17: Motor Vehicle Accident (MVA) Fatality Impacting First Responders and Bystander Witnesses

Case Study #18: MVA Fatality	Type of Contact or Incident	# Contacts	Hours Committed by FRCP Team	Initiating Dept.	Other Agencies Involved	Acuity Level of Service for Chaplain	Estimated $ Value, Based on Hours
Day of Event	Crisis Call (1 GCI)	12	3	Local Fire Dept.	EMS, Highway Patrol, FCSO	High	3 hours @ $125 per hour = $375
Day after Event	Meeting with Bystanders	2	2	Fire Dept.		Moderate	2 hours @ $125 per hour = $250
TOTAL	3	14	5	4		Median = High	$625

- Recruiting and retaining volunteers is an ongoing need. Newly documented evidence showing the increased risks of cancer among firefighters also exacerbates the dangers inherent in being a firefighter. See Appendix 4 for other critical FR tools, resources and links.

Case Study #18: Suicide Attempt on Hospital Campus

One of the hospital's Security Supervisor's contacted the Program Director informing him of a suicide attempt that had just occurred near one of the campus parking decks where a former patient with a suicidal history had threatened to jump prior to being pulled to safety. The supervisor's proactive call was made to ensure that all the officers involved and affected by this successful rescue attempt received the post-incident support they deserved. Two FRC Team members were deployed to a planned meeting for the security officers on the same day of this incident.

Lessons Learned from Case #18

- This incident should give pause to the public and all other hospital staff who may fail to appreciate the many varied stressors of Security Officers. While they do not consider their role to be one of enforcement, their presence is vital to ensuring the safety of all persons in the medical center environment (patients, staff, students, visitors). Achieving this task 24/7 requires a sophisticated level of communications and the capacity to quickly cover an expansive area that is immensely complex and challenging to navigate.

- In addition, Security Officers work daily in one of the most diverse environments imaginable. The influx of visitors alone into the campus can number in the thousands.

- As is typically experienced by First Responders in the larger community, visitors and staff in the medical center environment routinely depend on Security Officers to address a wide array of issues, ranging from visitors simply asking for direc-

In addition, Security Officers work daily in one of the most diverse environments imaginable. The influx of visitors alone into the campus can number in the thousands.

In this sense, the challenges facing the Security Officers far exceed those of many municipal police departments that are also smaller in size.

tions or staff seeking in-service safety training. However, a Security Officer's job can become dangerous and intensely stressful within minutes when dealing with an assaultive, violent visitor or patient, or rushing to an emergency as described in this case involving a suicidal individual.

- Therefore, a high level of training and vigilance is required of Security Officers to maintain the safety and routine functioning of the medical center. In this sense, the challenges facing the Security Officers far exceed those of many municipal police departments that are also smaller in size.

- This case highlights just one of many critical incidents that can occur in such a complex organization. Its emotional impact was obvious especially on the less experienced officers who had never dealt with a suicide attempt.

- The incident was rife with risks for both the responding Security Officers and for the suicidal individual. A safe rescue plan had to be quickly devised that would save the individual while also protecting the officers who could have easily fallen with the individual, or been pulled down by the individual, had the plan failed, causing serious injury or death to multiple persons.

- A typical post-incident response to even a successful rescue is one of emotional and physical exhaustion. Reliving the incident, imagining what could have gone wrong and fearing a recurrence are also common reactions that leave anxiety levels elevated for those officers who must soon return to duty.

- This incident was also made more complicated and stressful by witnesses due to the highly public location at a busy time of day.

- The normal chronic stressors inherent in doing the work of a Security Officer alongside the critical incident stress accompanying such a traumatic experience underscore why fitness for duty is imperative. The FRC Team has provided wellness and resiliency training for the Security Officers to address this need.

- As a unique subset of essential workers in the medical center, Security Officers deserve special recognition and appreciation for faithfully executing their duties during the unprecedented challenges of COVID-19 as they, along with other First Responder groups, struggle to hire and retain staff and contend with an ever-changing set of conditions in their highly complex work environment.

- The rapid connection between the Security Officers and the FRC Team regarding this incident would not have been possible without the pre-incident education, networking and trust-building between the two groups. The FRC Team also has a rich history of working with the Security Officers whenever First Responders killed in the LOD throughout the region are brought to the medical center for autopsy and later escorted home by their peers. While all of the hospital chaplains are a resource to the Security Officers, the FRC Team has essentially adopted them as part of the

Case Study #18: Suicide Attempt on Hospital Campus

Case Study #18: Suicide Attempt on Hospital Campus	Type of Contact or Incident	# Contacts	Hours Committed by FRCP Team	Initiating Dept.	Other Agencies Involved	Acuity Level of Service for Chaplain	Estimated $ Value, Based on Hours
Day of Event	Crisis Call	20	3	Hospital Security	EMS, Fire Dept., WSPD	High	3 hours @ $125 per hour = $375
Days after Event	Meeting	3 (GCI)	2	Hospital Security		Moderate	2 hours @ $200 per hour = $400
TOTAL	2	23	5			Median =	$775

It is critical for readers to note that a LODD, the death of a peer, especially a violent death, is ranked as the worst of possible critical incidents First Responders ever face over the course of their careers.

broader family of First Responders whose jobs predispose them to unique stressors and at times, heavy sensory exposure. To ensure immediate access to the FRC Team, all of the Security Officers have the FRC Team's cell numbers and team email to contact the team at all hours for both work-related and personal problems.

Case Study #19: Sergeant Mickey Hutchens' Law Enforcement LODD

It is critical for readers to note that a LODD, the death of a peer, especially a violent death, is ranked as the worst of possible critical incidents First Responders ever face over the course of their careers.

This unique case study is a very personal account of the impact that a LODD of a law enforcement officer can have upon the surviving family, a department and an entire community. According to Chris Cosgriff, Founder of the online Officer Down Memorial Page, "When a police officer is killed, it's not an agency that loses an officer, it's an entire nation."

Beth Hutchens is the widow of Sgt. Mickey Hutchens. Sgt. Hutchens, a 27-year veteran of the Winston-Salem Police Department (WSPD), was killed in the LOD on October 12, 2009, at 50 years of age. More details about his LODD can be found online.[10]

Beth retired from her work at Wake Forest University as a departmental administrator in 2010. She also worked at the LAPD as a Telecommunicator before moving to Winston-Salem, where she also served as a Telecommunicator at the WSPD.

Beth was interviewed by the authors on September 14 and 28, 2021. Below is her family's story with "lessons learned" woven into the narrative.

The day of the incident, Beth learned of an officer down call involving two officers at the Bojangles Restaurant on Peters Creek Parkway, located in Mickey's territory. She finally called the secretary in Internal Affairs, someone who knew Mickey well from his having previously worked there, and the secretary started crying. It was then that Beth knew that Mickey had been badly hurt. From the moment Beth arrived at AHWFB until the time of Mickey's eventual death, her family along with WSPD staff and other First Responder friends and colleagues kept a vigil at or near his bedside. There was an outpouring of community support.

Beth allowed open visitation to anyone in the WSPD who wanted a chance to be with Mickey and a select group of other individuals (a total of almost 300 people) to visit when Mickey was in the ICU and facing a grim prognosis. This processional of newly minted LEOs paid honor to Sgt. Hutchens, but were also acutely reminded of the dangers of the profession they had just entered.

As death grew imminent, Beth described having a real disconnect with Mickey's body, feeling as if his spirit had already departed. As a deeply spiritual person, Beth was consoled by her belief that it was Mickey's time to die and go to heaven.

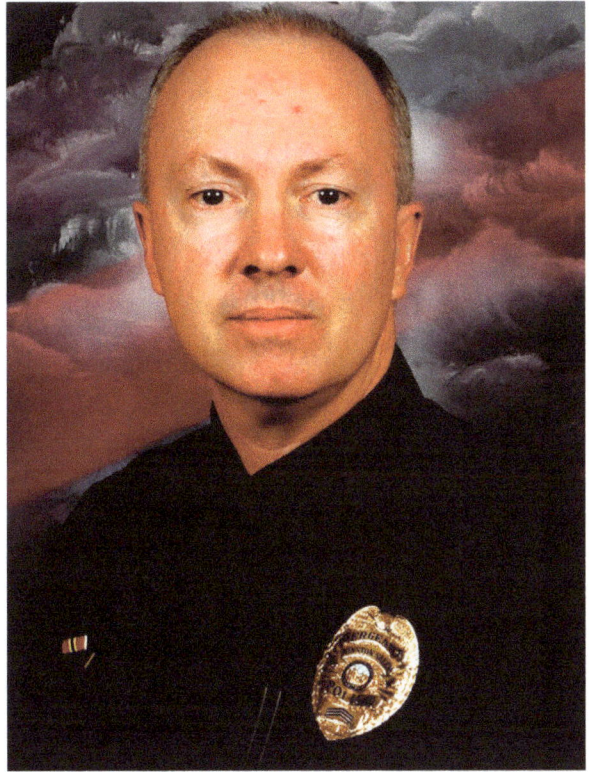

Fallen Officer Sergeant "Mickey" Gray Hutchens

Chaplain Davis, who was the FCSO Chaplain at the time, was asked by Beth to speak with a local pastor whose presence made Beth uncomfortable due to some family history with the pastor's church. The pastor complied with this request and understood that in times of trauma that unwelcome visitors, including even well-intentioned individuals, can inadvertently exacerbate a family's grief and potentially traumatize them further by violating a family's wishes and/or privacy.

After Mickey's death, Leah (Beth and Mickey's adult daughter) had an opportunity to vent her anger at the killer's wife, explaining that it was Leah's father who was killed. The killer's ex-wife lived in their community in Yadkin County (although the family did not know her) and had repeatedly told people that she was glad her ex-husband was dead. Leah explained that, although the killer's ex-wife was glad about this turn of events, Mickey's daughter and family were not happy for their loss.

It is critical that survivor families receive competent support. When Leah made the decision to seek counseling, she was surprised that the counselor cried, and she never went back to that counselor, finding it useless to her healing. This is not atypical since many counselors, in both the private sector and EAPs, do not understand the nature of traumatic grief, particularly the kind associated with a violent LODD and its overwhelming and life-changing impact on the survivor family, the entire First Responder agency and the community at large.

Beth, knowing that LODDs are especially hard on families with young children, counts herself blessed, as her children were in their early 20s at the time of their father's death.

Like the thousands of other spouses in fallen officer families, Beth's grief has been and continues to be triggered by other losses and trauma occurring throughout the First Responder community both locally, statewide and nationally. Given those stressors, 2020-21 may be remembered as one of the most dangerous times to be in law enforcement, not just in terms of the risks of physical injury, but also the combined risks for poor quality of life during one's career and even into retirement.

Beth describes how fallen officers' families, and particularly the surviving spouses feel stigmatized, not so much because of what happened to them, but by how others perceive and treat them. Every LODD heightens the sense of vulnerability for all officers and their families. The most dangerous risks of the job are on full display for all to see. Proximity to this intense grief and the bereaved themselves is discomforting to those who deny this vulnerability. For that reason, Beth has found that while she's been a great comfort to many families, she's aware that others have seen her as "the black crow of death," an older widow of a fallen officer whose presence and powerful story makes some law enforcement leaders uncomfortable.

Beth stated that Mickey's department later stopped asking her to talk to officers, because of her honesty in addressing the realities of LOD injuries and LODD. She felt stigmatized by some department members because her presence and strong personality afflicted the comfortable who didn't want to talk about the risks of being a LEO.

In Beth's case, one consolation in dealing with Mickey's death is that the perpetrator, who fatally shot her husband and wounded Officer Daniel Clark, was then killed by Officer Clark after he was wounded. The perpetrator's death eliminated what would surely have been a long and arduous trial, taxing many resources in the criminal justice system (CJS) and compounding the family's grief due to years of appeals and parole hearings. It also helped that Beth knew many staff at the WSPD and was a strong advocate for herself and her family.

Case Study #19: Sergeant Mickey Hutchens' Law Enforcement Officer LODD

Case Study #19: Sgt. Mickey Hutchens' LODD	Type of Contact or Incident	# Contacts	Hours Committed by FRCP Team	Initiating Dept.	Other Agencies Involved	Acuity Level of Service for Chaplain	Estimated $ Value, Based on Hours
Day of Event	Crisis Call	50	6	FCSO	EMS	High	6 hours @ $125 per hour = $750
Day after Event	Meeting	25	4	FCSO		Moderate	4 hours @ $200 per hour = $800
Weeks after Event	Support	100	8			Moderate	8 hours @ $125 per hour = $1000
One Year after Event	Follow-up Calls	5	2			Low	2 hours @ $125 per hour = $250
TOTAL	4	180	20			Median = Moderate	$2800

Other events in Beth's life proved that no trauma happens in a vacuum. Beth had a house fire in 2014, a week before the fifth anniversary of Mickey's death and her mother died the week after. A year later Beth was diagnosed with breast cancer.

Quicker Notification in the Event of LOD Injuries and LODD

In the chaos and media attention that often follow serious LOD injuries and most certainly LODDs, command level personnel must focus on the expeditious in-person notifications of the next of kin, especially the spouse. The trauma associated with the incident is made far worse for the family when there are delays or incomplete information or if the spouse or any other family member must seek out the information by making phone calls.

Today, social media with its potential to inform, or, in some cases, misinform an entire community, if not the nation, has added an even greater sense of time urgency to the notification of family members to respect their dignity and privacy. Hearing news of an officer involved shooting (OIS) or an officer down call over a police scanner also incites panic in the law enforcement family and only intensifies the need to receive accurate in-person information from the appropriate agency personnel (agency head, officer's supervisor, chaplain, among others).

The fear and panic incited in other spouses when the death is occurring in real time and the children and families hear about it is strong; many live each day dreading they might get the "call." Beth never worried about Mickey on calls because he had good judgment. Her prior work history also gave her a better understanding of the WSPD and the First Responder network.

Every agency has or should have policy-defined protocols outlining in detail how to address LODDs and all of the actions and procedures necessitated by such a loss. These include immediately assigning an advocate to the survivor spouse and family to help them attend to a range of tasks, particularly time-sensitive matters such as funeral arrangements, but also critical discussions concerning pensions and LODD benefits.

Organizations like C.O.P.S. encourage law enforcement officers and other First Responders to use some form of a Personal Information template that each agency can customize.[11]

This booklet can be used by officers to safely compile, update and secure critical personal information, such as insurance policies and beneficiaries, financial holdings, account passwords, etc., all of which can be immensely helpful to their families, saving them from unnecessary work and potential embarrassment if information is inaccurate or out of date. The confidential information should also include the officer's detailed wishes if killed in the LOD so that both the family and the impacted agency can appropriately honor the officer's service.

Concrete Help

Everyone says they will be there for you at the funeral. Two weeks later, everyone disappears. The family's grief endures long after the public mourning by the impacted agency and the community ends. What can be perceived by families as excessive attention in the days following a LODD quickly dissipates. Friends, neighbors and even church members also often don't know what to say or how to help. It would be better if people would not repeatedly ask the exhausted spouse and immediate loved ones "How are you?" but rather "What can I help you with?" Answering the latter question requires far less energy for the survivor spouse and quickly conjures up a laundry list of tasks and errands that must be addressed. Most importantly, it addresses the family's practical needs and empowers the helpers to actively focus on concrete, doable tasks, which assists with healthy grieving.

Institutional Impact

A LODD doesn't just scar a family, but impacts a whole agency and multiple communities. These impacts are further amplified and reverberate across the nation, demonstrating the dense and close networks that bond all law enforcement organizations. It's also critical to note that within each agency the trauma of a

Everyone says they will be there for you at the funeral. Two weeks later, everyone disappears. The family's grief endures long after the public mourning by the impacted agency and the community ends.

LODD impacts not just sworn staff, but all personnel including civilians, working in highly skilled and critical areas such as Telecommunications, records, IT, administration, forensics, detention and many others.

LODD Impact on Survivor Family

Even the healthiest, most functioning survivor families can experience interfamily tensions during such a chaotic time brought on by a sudden, violent and premature death that can involve differences of opinion. These differences can cover a range of issues, such how to memorialize their loved one, handle decisions about money, insurance and legal decisions of a civil or criminal nature if the perpetrator goes to trial, then to prison. The life-changing and chronic nature of the stressors accompanying many of these challenges and the fear they generate should not be underestimated. Hence, it is critical in the emotional aftermath that survivor families make well-informed decisions and have the expert guidance and advocacy they need.

Survivor families also grieve differently. Spousal grief is very different from a child's grief and especially so for younger children. Similarly, the grief of siblings and that of the parents and grandparents of the fallen officer are unique. Parents and grandparents grieve the loss of a future when their child/grandchild who chose to serve and protect others is killed in the LOD. The grief reactions range from anger and even intense rage that can be targeted or diffuse (directed at the perpetrator or toward fighting the injustices of the bureaucracies involved), to withdrawal and depression, acknowledging that the future they anticipated has been stolen and a part of them has also died.

COVID-19 has impacted every aspect of how First Responder agencies function across the nation, including how agencies can appropriately memorialize the deaths of officers, both active and retired. Though they are traditionally highly public events, visitations and funerals during COVID-19, as mentioned previously, have been scaled back for safety reasons, greatly affecting how families, agencies and communities grieve the death of our public servants. Additionally, now that COVID-19 has been identified as the leading cause of law enforcement deaths for 2020 (followed closely by cardiovascular deaths), there have been discussions about how a COVID-19-related cause of death might be considered a LODD. This is a complex issue considering that nationwide surveys indicated at the time of this writing that close to half of all First Responders (perhaps our most critical frontline workers along with healthcare providers) were opposed to mandatory COVID-19 vaccinations even though their jobs continually put them, their own families, peers and the pubic they took an oath to serve and protect at risk daily.

Survivor families need validation of the losses accompanying a LODD and agencies should realize that families are all unique and, therefore, should not all be treated as if they are the same with respect to how they need to grieve and cope. Most important for agencies and communities to realize is that the family's needs are long-lasting and many survivors are in shock throughout the public mourning phase that follows a LODD, regardless of the cause of death. A First Responder chaplain can help agencies differentiate between the specialized, targeted care needed by the survivor family and the grieving process essential for the organization's health as each group struggles to assimilate and memorialize such a great loss. It is incumbent upon First Responder agency heads to understand that preserving and appropriately honoring the memory of every fallen officer is vitally important to the family but also for the health of the institution and community.

Every agency has its own way of memorializing its own fallen officers. Again, because all fallen officer families are unique, not all find these public displays helpful. Some feel they are done only out of obligation without any real feeling attached. There are also differences, both nationally and statewide, between Sheriff's Offices and Police Departments, regarding the numbers and frequency of LODDs. For example, in Forsyth County, the WSPD, with 18 LODDs listed on its memorial page, has had far more LODDs than the FCSO, which has eight LODDs listed on its page.[12]

The wreath laying ceremony for Mickey is held annually on October 12th, his end of watch (EOW) date, in front of the City

A First Responder chaplain can help agencies differentiate between the specialized, targeted care needed by the survivor family and the grieving process essential for the organization's health as each group struggles to assimilate and memorialize such a great loss.

The phenomenal cumulative work accomplished by the FRC Team (October 2018 through March 2021) includes 18,803 number of contacts and 6,515 hours committed, serving the agencies and staff of the FCSO, EMS, Fire, DSS, PH, Emergency Management and others. Specifically, 1,375 crisis calls have been attended.

of Winston-Salem's Public Safety Center. Other WSPD fallen officers are similarly honored on their EOW dates. Staying connected to the survivor families and acknowledgement of the death over the long run is important.

Measures/Impact

The FRC Team keeps internal notes about a variety of incidents and calls for service from a broad range of individuals and groups, using a template that provides a means for the team to recall specifics of the incident, process/debrief and plan for follow-up contact, which is almost always necessary or may be triggered by a call from a survivor or loved one.

Other measures for success include the following project outcomes and measurement. Quarterly reporting includes de-identified, aggregate reporting of number of total encounters (7,000 projected), stratifying by FCSO, EMS, Fire, DSS, Public Health or Faith Community persons served. Additionally, services are stratified by crisis calls, group intervention, education, service to retirees, staff follow up, community forums, planning events, wellness trainings, First Responder community meetings and governmental task forces, as well as funerals/visitations and end-of-life requests and duties.

Each quarter the FRCP submits a report to the granting agency within four weeks of the end of quarter. Additionally, an annual invoice outlining costs incurred during the grant period, along with a final annual report of metrics outlined above is provided.

Since the January 2, 2019, "turn on" date of the expanded service to all County employees, the FRC Team has been providing quarterly utilization reports to the County (specifically to HR) to provide metrics while respecting the confidentiality critical to the team's work.

The phenomenal cumulative work accomplished by the FRC Team (October 2018 through March 2021) includes 18,803 number of contacts and 6,515 hours committed, serving the agencies and staff of the FCSO, EMS, Fire, DSS, PH, Emergency Management and others. Specifically, 1,375 crisis calls have been attended. Categories of service include crisis calls, staff support, meetings/events, education, GCIs, wellness education and more. Approximate 42 formal GCIs have also been conducted in the timeframe specified above. Additionally, 2,095 team member only hours have been logged in internal work and meetings.

> The importance of a Chaplaincy program and how important the relationship is between an agency and the services of support and guidance that are received from a Chaplaincy program cannot be measured. In today's world, mental health needs continue to impact everyone to include the First Responders. The fact that we have a program is so important, but the fact that we have an aggressive program is life-changing to our agencies and more importantly our First Responders.
>
> **Gary Styers**
> *Deputy Chief Fire Marshall*

Specifically, crisis calls are triggered by emergent needs that require immediate attention/response and/or activation and mobilization, and often involve a multi-agency response (e.g., law enforcement, EMS and/or Fire). Education efforts are needs-driven and group-specific, on a range of topics (e.g., wellness, resiliency, stress management, new employee orientation or NEOs, informational sessions about the FRCP) and hours include time for both preparation and delivery. GCIs are strategic, time-sensitive, highly-confidential, on-site responses, provided upon request asap following critical or traumatic incidents. Meetings/events include various non-crisis gatherings (e.g., scheduled staff meetings for FCSO and other Forsyth County departments, retiree groups, ceremonies, graduations, special recognition/services). Attendance at these is CRITICAL for trust-building with staff.

Staff support combines the following sub-categories with this rank order being typical: staff coping with multiple kinds of grief, loss and transition compounded by other stressors, including

The FRC Team triages these requests which can range from a high-profile multi-agency mobilization (e.g. mass casualty incident or barricaded subject with hostages) to a more localized tragedy (e.g., death notification following an overdose or homicide or illness/death of a First Responder family member).

individual and/or family needs, follow-up, illness/hospitalization, bereavement and mental health referrals. Mental health referrals are the least frequent of stated needs/stressors, which is often attributable to expeditious and preventive intervention and support, provided in person and on scene by the FRCP Team, along with follow-up care that leads to crisis resolution).

Our annual number of encounters for FY19 was 6,343, FY20 was 8,254, while FY21 was 5,381. (COVID-19 restrictions required the team, with the exception of the Director, to be furloughed at least one-quarter time.)

In terms of evaluation, case study categories can reflect large chunks of the FRC Team's work. Triangulating that with monetizing hours of time spent may be useful. Reach/encounters with duration of time and number of total contacts are important.

In the past, the hospital's Spiritual Care Daily Activity Report (DAR) was an inefficient reporting method for the FRCP Team and even compounded the team's work. Reporting methods for First Responder chaplaincy don't fit into what works for conventional "inside the hospital walls" chaplaincy.

Reports are the team's means of accountability to Forsyth County without divulging identifiers, etc. All of the FRC Team follow-up interactions and incident tracking are done using phone calls, encrypted emails and protected documentation. In 2021, a comprehensive Excel spreadsheet tracking ALL of the team's work, not just the County piece, was developed for future documentation purposes.

As mentioned elsewhere, the FRC Team requests for service come from all First Responder groups as well as numerous other community partners, many of whom do not yet help fund the FRCP which is currently an AHWFB/Forsyth County collaboration, though a contract with the City of Winston-Salem is expected to expand the collaboration in 2022. These requests are often generated by direct phone calls to the FRC Team's emergency number by command level personnel and Telecommunicators. The FRC Team triages these requests which can range from a high-profile multi-agency mobilization (e.g. mass casualty incident or barricaded subject with hostages) to a more localized tragedy (e.g., death notification following an overdose or homicide or illness/death of a First Responder family member). However, it is typical for any First Responder, First Responder's family member, or any other citizen or resident, who has been referred to the FRC Team for help, to access the team by direct phone calls, texts or emails to the entire team or to individual team members.

As the FRC Team adds coverage for City employees to their scope of practice, it may need other reporting mechanisms. However, there are six quarters or one and a half years of reporting for the County, cumulatively reported below.

Compiled cumulative metrics of number of encounters, hours and benchmark dollar value of work done by the FRC Team in serving various agency stakeholders since October 2018, up to Q-4 FY2021 (June 30, 2021) reflects a stunning grand total of 18,803 encounters, 6,515 hours, valued at cost benchmarking $811,656.

For the FCSO, that work entailed 14,040 encounters and 5,248.5 hours, for EMS the count was 1,588 encounters and 586 hours, for the Fire Dept. that was 922 encounters and 231 hours, for DSS that was 554 encounters and 147 hours, and for Public Health that was 171 encounters and 64.5 hours.

Team Meetings

Total team hours including formal meetings and consults with other team members related to the provision of chaplaincy services were 2,095 for this time period. The average of team hours per quarter was 232.78.

Other Key Components of the FRC Team's Work Not Captured in Quarterly High Level Reporting

Despite these herculean process metrics, it is also worth noting that these utilization reports do not adequately capture in numbers alone several other key components of the team's work such as:

1. The team's vigilance and many hours spent communicating via countless emails, texts, phone calls during workdays, weekends, holidays and evenings in efforts to respond to

Despite these herculean process metrics, it is also worth noting that these utilization reports do not adequately capture in numbers alone several other key components of the team's work...

and support County employees, their families and trauma victims in the community.

2. The time spent by the team to maintain and disseminate (on average once/week) a "Hospital-Carelist" PDF that the team's Director has provided within the FCSO for over 27 years. This document requires continuous updating and contacts with key staff and families who have requested to be added to this list that encourages intra-agency peer support and empathy.

3. Time devoted to intensive ongoing training for the FRC Team—a minimum of six hours/month and often double this amount.

4. Additional contacts, i.e. referrals from other agencies inside and outside of Forsyth County; other speaking engagements, consultations with other care-providers, etc. As just one example, the FRC Team devoted approximately 15 hours, to a creative project that grew out of the County's Opioid Taskforce (Camp HEAL in 2018), illustrating that much of the team's community engagement quickly generates new initiatives and leads to invaluable collaborations addressing critical needs in our city and county.

5. It is nearly impossible to quantify the impact of or demands generated by critical incidents, which are very time and energy intensive and often have a very diffuse impact, taking a toll on multiple groups of survivors-victims-witnesses and First Responders. These highly disruptive incidents can require deployment to multiple locations, multiple interventions (over days, possibly weeks) with impacted groups, innumerable phone calls, follow-up care, referrals, allotted time for team debriefs, organizational reviews (also known as after-action reviews or hotwashes), etc.

6. Time challenges are imposed by documentation needs. These are exacerbated due to operating in a 24/7/365 on-call coverage environment, often in adverse circumstances in unconventional settings such as being on scene at a trau-

matic event versus operating in a conventional office with normal work hours.

7. Utilization reports also do not include all travel time moving between callouts, meetings, all area hospitals, homes and workplaces of County staff and other clients the team assists.

The FRC Team shares office space at AHWFB, the Forsyth County Public Safety Center (FCPSC) and has access to other County First Responder work locations which the Director defines more as landing zones than conventional office spaces. This is intentional so that the team does not concentrate its resources in one place and can always be highly adaptive and responsive to incoming needs. To achieve this goal, the team relies heavily on its work-issued technology, vigilantly monitoring individual iPhones to quickly access and share critical information to deploy into the community and use resources as strategically as possible.

The FRCP Team holds regular team meetings, biweekly and more often if needed, that include but are not limited to the following goals:

- Ongoing skills training with particular focus on crisis response and traumatic stress within First Responder communities.

- Case consultation, review and follow-up care with patients/clients.

- Team debriefings after critical interventions facilitated by the team.

- Preparing for a variety of upcoming educational events GCIs being offered to First Responder agencies and community groups.

- Community engagement, networking, collaborations.

- Documentation of team activities (one-on-one and group interventions, hospital visitation, emergency callouts during the day and after work hours, ongoing staff support, etc.).

- Managing/editing the on-call schedule to adapt to changing needs.

Funding Sources and Program Costs

The FRC Team salaries and benefits for the Director and two chaplains, as well as operational costs, phone and other communication devices and office space, computers and supplies, are covered by AHWFB. The County covers salary and fringe for one FTE chaplain and the FCSO provides one vehicle for use by the FRCP Director. Salary for the Director and three FTE Chaplains was ~$172,000 for FY21. Other program costs (e.g., uniforms, supplies, mileage, benefits) totaled roughly $328,000, for a grand total of $500,000.

External Leadership Valuing of the FRC Team's Work

Validation of the FRCP by First Responders were solicited via emails, comments, quotes, testimonials from approximately 50 persons who benefitted from the FRC Team's work through the decades, including different types of stakeholders. A total of eight persons responded (16% response rate).

A few key extracted quotes from these stakeholders have been positioned and shared earlier in side bars, strategically placed throughout this book. However, the full expression of these statements are found below, along with the name and title of the stakeholder.

I would consider the Chaplaincy Program probably one of, if not the most critical, programs that can be instituted for First Responders in any jurisdiction. The stressors, hatreds, divorces and suicides that are happening among First Responders...especially in today's world are alarming. We need help...we need support, whether we can admit it or not.

Lt. Jerry Hobbs, Retired
Forsyth County Sheriff's Office

There have been several inmates that have completed suicide over the years and the Chaplains will come in and be there for the officers that were involved in finding the inmates, cutting down inmates from hanging, trying to stop them from bleeding out, or just being involved in the situation. These are things that can be very stressful and even life changing for everyone involved. With the Chaplains being there to comfort and support, it is amazing to watch and experience. There has been a lot of negativity involving law enforcement for a while now and the Chaplains attending some meeting offering devotion and prayers has help keep our minds and spirits where they need to be. It is amazing how sometimes they say just what you need to hear, just when you need to hear it. I have come to know all of the Chaplains and very much appreciate all prayers, support and comfort they offer to not only us on the professional side, but on the personal life side as well. I have my own church I go to, and love the support I receive from my church, but it there are times professionally that it is more comfortable turning to a Chaplain because they understand the life of our profession.

Sergeant Lori Wood
Forsyth County Law Enforcement Detention Center

As the Fire Marshal of Forsyth County, my job comes with the responsibility of handling many different types of crises involving the public and First Responders. These crises can range from notifying a family of a loss of a loved one in the event of a fire to handling and supporting emergency services employee needs to include our partner First Responder agencies.

Thus, the importance of a Chaplaincy program and how important the relationship is between an agency and the services of support and guidance that are received from a Chaplaincy program cannot be measured. In today's world, mental health needs continue to impact everyone to include the First Responders. The fact that we have a program is so important, but the fact that we have an aggressive program is life-changing to our agencies and more importantly our First Responders.

Gary Styers
Deputy Chief Fire Marshal

While I consider myself fortunate that these things [work traumas] don't creep in on me daily, I know how important programs like these are. I can normally put these things in their box and file them away. But, having a support system is so very important in this area. Having someone like Glenn at the Sheriff's Office was great. If you didn't reach out to him first, he would reach out to you. Sometimes it may be nothing more than "Are you okay?" It is important to have a way to debrief, even if it is small. Sometimes you just have to refocus on your human side. It is important to know that someone who understands, cares about what you have seen and done. It's not normal for anyone to pick up pieces and parts of a body and put it in a bag. It's not normal to see a child eviscerated on an autopsy table. At the end of the day, we end up at home like everyone else eating dinner even though we have seen and done things that just aren't normal. We have to have each other's backs. You can't unburden these things with your spouses and loved ones because of confidentiality. I know first-hand how important it was to have a Chaplain on staff at the Sheriff's Office. You have to be a First Responder, but you are also human. You also have to remind yourself sometimes that you are human and not a work machine.

I see so much more now about how important mental health is in this type of profession. It seems like the tough guy stigma is slowly evaporating, which I am glad of and I credit a lot of this to awareness and "the First Responder for the First Responder.

Sean Reid
Medicolegal Death Investigator
Atrium Health Wake Forest Baptist (AHWFB)

During any given day or night, early or late, it doesn't matter. Someone is there to respond. It may be a phone call; it may be a personal visit. But they are there.

One Easter Sunday at about 7:00AM, I got a phone call from an employee that I supervised. Her brother had just been killed in a plane crash. I consoled her the best I could. Then I called Glenn Davis. BAM, he sprang into action. Getting this woman much needed attention that she needed. It was immediate. Not the next day. IMMEDIATE.

Sometimes where you work doesn't matter. I have a dear friend of 35+ years that was in the hospital with COVID-19. His spirit was broken. No one could go see him and at times he wasn't texting or answering the phone. I emailed the chaplains ... BAM ... I get a phone call from Dana Patrick. She understood that my friend wasn't a Sheriff. It didn't matter. She knew I was worried and therefore she knew she had to act and did she ever. She called my friend twice, letting me know each time that he was hanging in there the best he could. She was also praying for him. A week or so later, one of the finest attorneys in the state of NC also was hanging on to life by a thread with COVID-19. I emailed the chaplains and BAM, almost immediately got a response that they were praying for him....

When my grandson was born in Greensboro, N.C and was two days old, he had to go to Brenner's with a high fever. I met my wife and daughter there. When the little guy needed a spinal tap, I called Glenn Davis … BAM … he showed up moments later. Not hours. Moments. He hugged me in the hallway then came into the room and prayed with my daughter, wife and I. It didn't stop there. Aaron Eaton also came by and prayed with us. Weeks after that, Aaron was coming by my office to make sure the little man was doing well….

These are just a few examples of probably countless times these chaplains have stepped up in much needed situations. They are more than just a resource. They care. They are friends. They are a shoulder to cry on or a smile when you need it most.

When my wife and I were going to be married, the only name that came to mind was Glenn Davis. It was both of our second marriages and we wanted something small. Eloping basically. Glenn met with us a few times for some pre-marriage counseling and in the end, we were married in our own living room wearing shorts and flip-flops. We were the luckiest couple on the planet. Not only were we getting married, but we were going to be forever tied to Glenn as well, something that means so much more to us than anyone will ever know.

It doesn't matter where I am or what I am doing. If Glenn Davis, Dana Patrick, Aaron Eaton or Jeff Vogler and I make eye contact, there is always time for a quick chat. It doesn't matter what the conversation is. Sometimes they can see when someone is troubled and know they need an ear.

They are all nothing short of amazing.

Sergeant Roger Dunlap
Forsyth County Sheriff's Office

EMS got involved with Glenn Davis through the FCSO. Glenn's name became synonymous with being the "go-to Guy" when they needed any chaplaincy service. In 2016, MIH (Mobile Integrated Healthcare) team was developed by Forsyth County Emergency Services. This Community Paramedic team responds to many different types of calls but mostly assists with behavioral health, substance use and individuals who have become reliant on the 911 system for healthcare. They connect people with resources to address their current needs, like help after the unexpected death of a child. I and my team always trusted Glenn and his team and vice versa. It got to the point where, if MIH ran a bad scene, we would have kids or adults who were exposed to deaths or crime scenes (often caused by the opioid crisis) and we would call Glenn and his team to come out and be unbiased, non-judgmental, supportive and caring contact person for all persons involved, regardless of their beliefs. Glenn and his team turned into that "shoulder" to lean on that people needed. Glenn and his team often can do follow up with those in the community and that is so important. First responders have often been discouraged from establishing that continuity of care. Glenn's team are on the scene as FaithHealth caregivers and provide that for the families.

Then I thought, well, we need that type of care for our own team. When we are exposed to all those deaths and trauma, we need support, too. So, Glenn and his team became that support for the Forsyth County Emergency Services, especially in terms of all the opioid deaths that MIH team members have seen. Glenn never says "No." I don't know how he does it.

Glenn's team then became the "go-to" team for how to deescalate people after traumatic events and provide reality-based care that works. It is so valuable.

One of my team is really into CISM and Glenn says, well, it's a good model, but we have to make it work with the local community. Glenn taught us about what actually works in the community in which we live. Glenn's team can tie us into churches, chaplains or other staff at AHWFB or Novant and other critical resources and persons who can help. He and his team are truly compassionate people who have an amazing ability to interact in a supportive and humble way that allows people who have just experienced an unimaginable event to open up and seek help. I and my team built a peer support program with Glenn's guidance. Chris Nichols who runs that program day-to-day, under my oversight, but it truly was developed, based on Glenn's expertise.

Glenn and I attended a DHHS convention about how to engage the faith community in the opioid crisis, which was held in Washington DC and one of the keynote speakers was the head of the CDC, Dr. Robert R. Redfield. Glenn and I were able to speak to groups of professionals from around the country who were both from the faith community and the substance use and medical treatment communities. Participants were all very excited about the model we had built where my team of First Responder paramedics utilize Glenn's chaplains to support and connect individuals to resources and follow up with them for continued questions and care needs that arise. Glenn's team being part of the initial event and being able to follow families through their journey of grief and healing is a service that is immeasurably important.

Captain Brent Motsinger
Community Paramedic
Mobile Integrated Healthcare

Twelve years ago, my husband who was a 28-year veteran of WSPD was shot and died five days later. I am anxious that that experience be used to help others in the future.

I know that there is so much that could be learned to help others from an empirical study of families of fallen officers.... For now I am excited about what you are doing now and would love to help you out in any way.

Beth Hutchens
Widow of Fallen Officer

Themes Noted from External Stakeholder Quotations/Story Cited Above about the FRC Team

- Provide constant and sustained support and comfort.

- Embedded chaplain model (within the extended First Responder family).

- Proactive "Search and Find" chaplaincy model approach.

- Understanding context of the various First Responder cultures and professions.

- Constant support and sounding board in coping with highly traumatic and stressful work events.

- Confidentiality and safety of encounters, plus non-judgmental stance.

- Importance of the FRC Team's high level of accessibility and ability to link to extensive mental health networks.

- Focus on being human versus a robotic First Responder.

- Constantly available in terms of accessibility and immediacy.

- Care extended to First Responder families when a family member is ill or to neighbors, colleagues and friends who experience tragedy, extending to conducting funerals, but also available for celebratory events, like weddings, promotions, retirements, births of children/grandchildren.

- Long-term support is especially important to the survivor families of fallen First Responders.

- Learning/training, helping other First Responders and families in the aftermath of LODDs and many other losses and transitions.

Acknowledgements

We wish to give deep thanks to FRC Team members Dana Patrick, MDiv, Aaron Eaton, MDiv, and Jeff Vogler, MDiv, for their dedicated service and invaluable contributions to the lives of First Responders and their families, the success of the FRCP and its future sustainability. Also we appreciate their insights, materials and help in crafting this document.

Appreciation is also extended to Beth Hutchens for her transparent and thoughtful sharing about the LODD of her husband, WSPD Sergeant Mickey Gray Hutchens and its impact on her family, the community and agency he served. Brian Davis, DMin and Anita Holmes, JD, MPH offered general stylistic comments to this piece. We are also grateful to the North Carolina Baptist Foundation for their support. Lastly, we'd like to thank all the stakeholders who contributed their quotes about the value of the FRC Team for this book, as well as all First Responders across the globe, who give all their energy, passion and compassion in serving and protecting all of us.

Endnotes

1 Stanley, I.H., Horn, M.A., Hagan, C.R., Joiner, T.E., 2015. Career prevalence and correlates of suicidal thoughts and behaviors among firefighters. J. Affect. Disord. 187, 163–171. http://dx.doi.org/10.1016/j.jad.2015.08.007

2 Hegg-Deloye S, Brassard P, Jauvin N, Prairie J, Larouche D, Poirier P, Tremblay A, Corbeil P. Current state of knowledge of post-traumatic stress, sleeping problems, obesity and cardiovascular disease in paramedics. Emerg Med J. 2014 Mar;31(3):242-7. doi: 10.1136/emermed-2012-201672. Epub 2013 Jan 12.

3 *See* https://www.wbfj.fm/painful-memories-wednesday-is-the-25th-anniversary-of-the-1988-michael-hayes-shootings-along-old-salisbury-road

4 *See* https://www.cbsnews.com/news/3-fans-killed-at-indy-race *and* https://us.motorsport.com/nascar-cup/news/charlotte-pedestrian-walkway-collapses/1806210

5 *See* https://www.go2mro.com

6 *See* https://abcnews.go.com/US/30-years-27-died-worst-drunk-driving-crash/story?id=55119258

7 *See* https://www.odmp.org

8 *See* https://www.cbsnews.com/news/covid-19-is-nations-biggest-cop-killer-officers-vaccine-resistant

9 *See* https://www.nfpa.org/News-and-Research/Data-research-and-tools/Emergency-Responders/US-fire-department-profile *and* https://apps.usfa.fema.gov/registry/summary

10 *See* https://www.cityofws.org/1181/Sergeant-Mickey-Gray-Hutchens

11 *See* https://irp-cdn.multiscreensite.com/ac5c0731/files/uploaded/Personal%20Information%20Form.pdf. *See also their websites, both national and state:* https://www.concernsofpolicesurvivors.org *and* https://www.nccops.net.

12 *See* https://www.cityofws.org/1374/Memorials *and* https://www.co.forsyth.nc.us/sheriff/officer_memorials.aspx

Appendix 1

Glossary of Commonly Used Terms

Chain of Command (COC)

Chaplain—A clinically-trained staff chaplain employed by AHWFB or chaplain in training, also known as a chaplain resident or chaplain fellow, providing spiritual care, crisis intervention services and education to a broad range of First Responders, government agencies/departments and individuals and families throughout the community, whose lives have been impacted by trauma of all kinds. All chaplains comprising the FRC Team report to the FRCP Director.

Clinical Pastoral Education (CPE)—Professional post-graduate education for clergy based upon a dynamic experiential process of learning from living human documents, oneself, others, and especially persons in various life crises. CPE is founded upon the premise that pastoral care and counseling must provide ministry to the whole person.

Concerns of Police Survivors (C.O.P.S.)—National organization (with state branches) that provides advocacy and support to families of officers who have died.

Confidential Personal Affairs Booklet—A booklet developed by the Program Director for FCSO, but patterned after similar templates provided by C.O.P.S. and other organizations. Its purpose is to assist First Responders who voluntarily wish to collect and organize confidential personal/financial or other information for their loved ones in the event of the participating staff member's serious injury or death. See endnote 11 on page 142 for a link to the C.O.P.S. Personal Information Form.

Crisis calls—Defined emergent needs requiring immediate attention/response and/or activation and mobilization of the FRC Team to one or more scenes. Some incidents are "roving" meaning that a crisis such as a death can necessitate timely interventions or traumatic message notifications with multiple persons at multiple locations. Many crisis calls are protracted, lasting several hours, depending on the complexity of a law enforcement investigation, dynamics of the bereaved family, and/or the extensive impact of an incident on multiple communities of people, such as a multi-casualty event in a neighborhood, at a school or business. Note that a crisis call initiated by one agency almost always involves a multi-agency response (including, but not limited to, law enforcement, EMS and Fire) requiring immediate attention or response and/or activation and mobilization.

Critical Incident—Any traumatic event with the capacity to cause physical or psychological injury and impair functioning. Such an event is often beyond the realm of a person's normal experiences and has the potential to elicit unusually strong emotional reactions which can potentially interfere with the affected individual's ability to function either at the time of the incident or later. While the public and all non-First Responder groups are at some risk of experiencing critical incidents, First Responders are much more susceptible to more frequent exposure due to the nature of their work. Examples of critical incidents within First Responder populations may include but are not limited to: Line of duty death (LODD), line of duty (LOD) injury, officer involved shooting (OIS), suicide of a coworker, other non-LOD traumatic death/injury of a coworker or family member, mass casualty event, death of a child, death notification, prolonged failed rescue attempt, traumatic event in which the victim is known to the First Responder, termination of employment, protracted internal affairs investigation, any event perceived to be threatening or potentially threatening to the safety of a staff member which might potentially induce psychological and/or physical responses and seriously impair life functioning and/or work performance.

Critical Incident Stress (CIS)—Intense stress resulting from an individual observing or experiencing a traumatic or critical incident. CIS may be experienced vicariously by indirect exposure to another individual's traumatic event and emotions. It refers to acute or delayed post-incident stress reactions or symptoms an individual may exhibit following exposure to or participation in a critical incident. These signals of distress, exhibited after a critical incident, are typically observed in five domains: physical, cognitive, emotional, behavioral, and spiritual.

Critical Incident Stress Debriefing (CISD)—Describes the most complex and formal intervention, the seven-stage debriefing process, as just one of a constellation of interventions within the scope of CISM.

Critical Incident Stress Management (CISM)—The comprehensive crisis intervention system developed by the International Critical Incident Stress Foundation (ICISF) that comprises the universally adopted standards of care for many First Responders, the military and other organizations within the private and public sectors.

Critical Incident Reaction—Individuals react differently to CIS, depending upon factors such as the type of threat, the intensity and duration of the sensory exposure accompanying the incident. Individual past experiences, coping skills, concurrent stressors, as well as the social and agency support systems available before, during and after the incident can affect the impact of the incident on the individual(s) involved.

Forsyth County Emergency Services (FCES) includes both Fire and EMS (Emergency Medical Services)

Forsyth Jail and Prison Ministry (FJPM)—Non-profit ministry that has a long history of serving inmate populations and their families within Forsyth County and maintains a regular presence inside of the Forsyth County Law Enforcement Detention Center.

Group Crisis Intervention (GCI)—A GCI, also known as a defusing, is one of many crisis intervention models that is strategic, efficient, highly applicable, time-sensitive and always confidential. It involves on-site response, provided upon request as soon as possible following critical or traumatic incidents usually within eight to 12 hours of an incident's occurrence.

Hospital Care List (HCL)—This document has been used by the Program Director throughout his chaplaincy career and is currently used by the FRC Team. It is carefully edited at least weekly and distributed via email by the FRC Team to the entire FCSO extended family, including retirees, for the purpose of sharing a wide range of information (e.g., hospitalizations, pending surgeries, funeral arrangements and celebratory news such as the birth of children and grandchildren, etc.). Information is shared only with expressed permission of each First Responder or his/her family. Due to the size of the First Responder extended family and the scope of needs, this document requires continuous updating and communications with key staff and families who have requested to be added to this list. The HCL focuses on the care of the FCSO family and also encourages intra-agency peer support and empathy.

International Association of Firefighters (IAFF) www.iaff.org

Line of Duty Death (LODD)—Death of a First Responder while on active duty or engaged in agency functions.

Officer Down Memorial Page (ODMP)—www.odmp.org. The National Law Enforcement Officers Memorial (NLEOM at https://nleomf.org/memorial) is the nation's monument to LEOs who have died in the LOD. Dedicated on October 15,

1991, the Memorial honors federal, state and local law enforcement officers who have made the ultimate sacrifice for the safety and protection of our nation and its people.

Post-Traumatic Stress Disorder (PTSD)—A debilitating mental health condition most often triggered by exposure to a highly stressful incident and often accompanied by flashbacks, severe anxiety, nightmares and persistent, disturbing thoughts and memories associated with the incident.

Sensory Exposure—Refers to the degree of proximity, intensity, duration and type of exposure to which all of the primary senses (sight, hearing, touch, taste, smell) and other senses of temperature, pain, body awareness, time perception and equilibrium may be affected by an individual's exposure to a traumatic event.

Survivors-Victims-Witnesses—Anyone, including First Responders or civilians, having the potential to be traumatized physically or psychologically by some degree of sensory exposure as a result of witnessing or being in close proximity to the critical incident itself or relationally close to the incident through a family member, neighbor, work colleague or peer.

Appendix 2

Key Academic References About First Responder Stress and Health Status

1. Norton K. Responding to a suicide death: The role of First Responders. Death Stud. 2017 Nov-Dec; 41(10): 639-647. doi: 10.1080/07481187.2017.1335550. Epub 2017 Jun 9. PMID: 28598715.

2. Piñar-Navarro E, Cañadas-De la Fuente GA, González-Jiménez E, Hueso-Montoro C. Anxiety and strategies for coping with stress used by First Responders and out-of-hospital emergency health care staff before COVID-19. Emergencias. 2020 Sep;32(5):371-373. English, Spanish. PMID: 33006842.

3. Phung VH, Trueman I, Togher F, Orner R, Siriwardena AN. Community First Responders and responder schemes in the United Kingdom: systematic scoping review. Scand J Trauma Resusc Emerg Med. 2017 Jun 19;25(1):58. doi: 10.1186/s13049-017-0403-z. PMID: 28629382; PMCID: PMC5477292.

4. Liston C. Estimating Psychiatric Outcomes in First Responders. JAMA Netw Open. 2020 Sep 1;3(9):e2018678. doi: 10.1001/jamanetworkopen.2020. 18678. PMID: 32990733.

5. Kowalski C. Leadership of first-responders following trauma. J Bus Contin Emer Plan. 2019 Jan 1;13(1):81-90. PMID: 31462365.

6. Joyce S, Shand F, Lal TJ, Mott B, Bryant RA, Harvey SB. Resilience@Work Mindfulness Program: Results From a Cluster Randomized Controlled Trial With First Responders. J Med Internet Res. 2019 Feb 19;21(2):e12894. doi: 10.2196/12894. PMID: 30777846; PMCID: PMC6399574.

7. Jones S. Describing the Mental Health Profile of First Responders: A Systematic Review [Formula: see text]. J Am Psychiatr Nurses Assoc. 2017 May;23(3):200-214. doi: 10.1177/1078390317695266. Epub 2017 Feb 1. PMID: 28445653.

8. Haugen PT, McCrillis AM, Smid GE, Nijdam MJ. Mental health stigma and barriers to mental health care for First Responders: A systematic review and meta-analysis. J Psychiatr Res. 2017 Nov;94:218-229. doi: 10.1016/j.jpsychires.2017.08.001. Epub 2017 Aug 5. PMID: 28800529.

9. Lewis-Schroeder NF, Kieran K, Murphy BL, Wolff JD, Robinson MA, Kaufman ML. Conceptualization, Assessment, and Treatment of Traumatic Stress in First Responders: A Review of Critical Issues. Harv Rev Psychiatry. 2018 Jul/Aug;26(4):216-227. doi: 10.1097/HRP.0000000000000176. PMID: 29975339; PMCID: PMC6624844.

10. Stanley, I.H., Horn, M.A., Hagan, C.R., Joiner, T.E., 2015. Career prevalence and correlates of suicidal thoughts and behaviors among firefighters. J. Affect. Disord. 187, 163–171. http://dx.doi.org/10.1016/j.jad.2015.08.007.

11. Hegg-Deloye S, Brassard P, Jauvin N, Prairie J, Larouche D, Poirier P, Tremblay A, Corbeil P. Current state of knowledge of post-traumatic stress, sleeping problems, obesity and cardiovascular disease in paramedics. Emerg Med J.

2014 Mar;31(3):242-7. doi: 10.1136/emermed-2012-201672. Epub 2013 Jan 12.

12. DiGravio GM. Researchers find majority of fire and ambulance recruits overweight or obese [Internet]. 2009 [cited 2021Apr6]. Available from: https://news.harvard.edu/gazette/story/2009/03/researchers-find-majority-of-fire-and-ambulance-recruits-overweight-or-obese/.

13. Wilson D. An EMS Emergency: Sleep deprivation and fatigue [Internet]. 2015 [cited 2021Apr6]. Available from: https://www.emsworld.com/article/12135723/an-ems-emergency-sleep-deprivation-and-fatigue.

14. Jerome GJ, Lisman PJ, Dalcin AT, Clark A. Weight management program for First Responders: Feasibility study and lessons learned. Work. 2020;65(1):161-166. doi: 10.3233/WOR-193069. PMID: 31868723.

15. Smith DL, Graham E, Stewart D, Mathias KC. Cardiovascular Disease Risk Factor Changes Over 5 Years Among Male and Female US Firefighters. J Occup Environ Med. 2020 Jun;62(6):398-402. doi: 10.1097/JOM.0000000000001846. PMID: 32097285.

16. Kaipust CM, Jahnke SA, Poston WSC, Jitnarin N, Haddock CK, Delclos GL, Day RS. Sleep, Obesity, and Injury Among US Male Career Firefighters. J Occup Environ Med. 2019 Apr;61(4):e150-e154. doi: 10.1097/JOM.000000000000 1559. PMID: 30789448.

17. Gurevich KG, Poston WS, Anders B, Ivkina MA, Archangelskaya A, Jitnarin N, Starodubov VI. Obesity prevalence and accuracy of BMI-defined obesity in Russian firefighters. Occup Med (Lond). 2017 Jan;67(1):61-63. doi: 10.1093/occmed/kqw136. Epub 2016 Sep 30. PMID: 27694377.

18. Jahnke SA, Poston WS, Haddock CK, Jitnarin N. Obesity and incident injury among career firefighters in the central United States. Obesity (Silver Spring). 2013

Aug;21(8):1505-8. doi: 10.1002/oby.20436. Epub 2013 Jun 13. PMID: 23512940.

19. Fahs CA, Smith DL, Horn GP, Agiovlasitis S, Rossow LM, Echols G, Heffernan KS, Fernhall B. Impact of excess body weight on arterial structure, function, and blood pressure in firefighters. Am J Cardiol. 2009 Nov 15;104(10): 1441-5. doi.

20. Kales SN, Tsismenakis AJ, Zhang C, Soteriades ES. Blood pressure in firefighters, police officers, and other emergency responders. Am J Hypertens. 2009 Jan;22(1):11-20. doi: 10.1038/ajh.2008.296. Epub 2008 Oct 16. PMID: 18927545.

21. Yoo HL, Franke WD. Prevalence of cardiovascular disease risk factors in volunteer firefighters. J Occup Environ Med. 2009 Aug;51(8):958-62. doi: 10.1097/JOM.0b013e3181 af3a58. PMID: 19620889.10.1016/j.amjcard.2009.07.009. Epub 2009.

Appendix 3

Article in "Verbatim" about Chaplain Davis's early work in the Forsyth County Sheriff's Office (FCSO)

Verbatim was a bimonthly publication of the Department of Pastoral Care, North Carolina Baptist Hospitals, Inc. This article is reprinted here with permission.

Rev. Glenn Davis Works With Victims in a Specialized Setting

One night in the summmer of 1988, a man started shooting at cars on a rural road near Winston-Salem, NC. Before that night was over, he had killed four people and wounded three others.

But there were more than seven victims. What about their families, their friends, other people who were shot at but not hit, people who lived in the area of the shooting, and law enforcement officers and emergency medical service workers on the scene? They were also victims, the surviving (and often overlooked) victims of crime.

The Rev. Glenn Davis is the Chaplain and Victim Counselor with the Forsyth County Sheriff's Department Victim Assistance Program. He does crisis intervention and referral with survivors of homicide, suicide and other traumatic death victims; and victims of kidnapping, robbery and assault. "Even certain property crimes can have a devastating impact upon individuals and families," he says.

Davis has been with the program for four years, including when the only financial support came from grant funds. "There's no prototype for this work. It's exciting to be paving new ground. For people in clinical training, law enforcement is a wide-open field."

Davis trained at the School of Pastoral Care in 1979 and 1982, and completed a residency here from 1984–85. He did half his residency in the emergency room and intensive care. "These critical care areas were a special calling for me. That's where I felt most energized and most able to help," he explains. "More and more in the work I do, I see how valuable Pastoral Care training has been. I can't think of a better preparation to help me deal with such a diversity of crises while ministering to the whole person."

Chaplain on wheels

Many victims of crime are too traumatized to seek help, he says. "They often have no energy to pick up the phone and call. So I go to them. This isn't a 'wait and treat' model—it's more like 'search and find.'"

Although Davis has an office, he is usually out in the community. "I meet people at the scene of a tragedy, in their homes, in hospitals, the workplace—wherever we can get together." He is also on the road speaking to church groups and other organizations about how they can be more supportive of crime and trauma victims, and avoid re-victimizing those who are already hurting.

"Believing that the church can be the greatest support system for victims, I network with local clergy whenever possible. However, many times I am the pastor to those without a pastor. I'm a chaplain on wheels," he says.

Empowering victims

An important part of Davis' work is helping crime victims overcome a sense of powerlessness and depersonalization. "In this country's system of justice, the scales are tipped toward the defendant. People watch crime dramas on TV where all the bad guys go to jail, but in real life they are shocked to see their own offenders back on the street."

Many victims feel they are nothing but witnesses for the state, Davis says. "The personal nature of what was done to them, their homes, their families, seems to be overlooked. For example, the parents of a murdered child were warned not to cry during the trial proceedings, or they would be asked to leave the courtoom because they might 'prejudice the jury.'

"My job is to help empower victims so they can regain control after being re-victimized in situations like this."

Help for service providers

Working with law enforcement officers presents a special challenge. "Although officers are under a great deal of stress," Davis comments, "there has traditionally been a stigma attached to coming for help. Fortunately, this macho image in changing, but a lot still has to be unlearned."

Davis is also part of Special Operation Response Team (SORT) which provides "stress debriefings" with emergency services personnel to facilitate their recovery from critical incidents which can be traumatic for them. His office is located away from the Sheriff's Department, which offers more confidentiality for service providers and victims who need support.

National involvement

In addition to his local work, Davis is also a member of the National Organization for Victim Assistance (NOVA), a group which responds to national disasters. Over the years, he has participated as a volunteer on special NOVA crisis response teams sent to the sites of major disasters such as the Amtrak train wreck in Chase, MD, and the bus crash in Radcliff, KY. He led trainings and debriefings with affected communities, and met with clergy to help them prepare for handling the numerous spiritual questions that would arise in the aftermath of the disasters.

Support for caregivers

Davis realizes that caregivers like himself also need support. His own support system is an informal network of pastor friends, hospital friends, and other people he can pick up the phone and call. In addition, he receives support from Farmington Baptist Church in Farmington, NC, where he has been pastor for the last four years.

"I can leave the crisis mode and be with church family. I get nurturing and affection—it's a complete change for me. And it's a good reminder that what I am doing *is* a ministry."

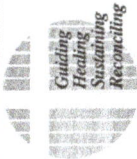

Rev. Glenn Davis Works With Victims in a Specialized Setting

One night in the summer of 1988, a man started shooting at cars on a rural road near Winston-Salem, N.C. Before that night was over, he had killed four people and wounded three others.

But there were more than seven victims. What about their families, their friends, other people who were shot at but not hit, people who lived in the area of the shooting, and law enforcement officers and emergency medical service workers on the scene? They were also victims, the surviving (and often overlooked) victims of crime.

The Rev. Glenn Davis is the Chaplain and Victim Counselor with the Forsyth County Sheriff's Department Victim Assistance Program. He does crisis intervention and referral with survivors of homicide, suicide and other traumatic death victims; and victims of kidnapping, robbery and assault. "Even certain property crimes can have a devastating impact upon individuals and families," he says.

Davis has been with the program for four years, including when the only financial support came from grant funds. "There's no prototype for this work. It's exciting to be paving new ground. For people in clinical training, law enforcement is a wide-open field."

Davis trained at the School of Pastoral Care in 1979 and 1982, and completed a residency here from 1984-86. He did half his residency in the emergency room and intensive care. "These critical care areas were a special calling for me. That's where I felt most energized and most able to help," he explains. "More and more in the work I do, I see how valuable Pastoral Care training has been. I can't think of a better preparation to help me deal with such a diversity of crises while ministering to the whole person."

Chaplain on wheels

Many victims of crime are too traumatized to seek help, he says. "They often have no energy to pick up the phone and call. So I go to them. This isn't a 'wait and treat' model — it's more like 'search and find.'"

Although Davis has an office, he is usually out in the community. "I meet people at the scene of a tragedy, in their homes, in hospitals, the workplace — wherever we can get together." He is also on the road speaking to church groups and other organizations about how they can be more supportive of crime and trauma victims, and avoid re-victimizing those who are already hurting.

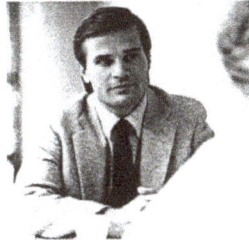

The Rev. Glenn Davis, M.Div.

"Believing that the church can be the greatest support system for victims, I network with local clergy whenever possible. However, many times I am the pastor to those without a pastor. I'm a chaplain on wheels," he says.

Empowering victims

An important part of Davis' work is helping crime victims overcome a sense of powerlessness and de-personalization. "In this country's system of justice, the scales are tipped toward the defendant. People watch crime dramas on TV where all the bad guys go to jail, but in real life they are shocked to see their own offenders back on the street."

Many victims feel they are nothing but witnesses for the state, Davis says. "The personal nature of what was done to them, their homes, their families, seems to be overlooked. For example, the parents of a murdered child were warned not to cry during the trial proceedings, or they would be asked to leave the courtroom because they might 'prejudice the jury.'

"My job is to help empower victims so they can regain control after being re-victimized in situations like this."

Help for service providers

Working with law enforcement officers presents a special challenge. "Although officers are under a

great deal of stress," Davis comments, "there has traditionally been a stigma attached to coming for help. Fortunately, this macho image is changing, but a lot still has to be unlearned."

Davis is also part of Special Operation Response Team (SORT) which provides "stress debriefings" with emergency services personnel to facilitate their recovery from critical incidents which can be traumatic for them. His office is located away from the Sheriff's Department, which offers more confidentiality for service providers and victims who need support.

National involvement

In addition to his local work, Davis is also a member of the National Organization for Victim Assistance (NOVA), a group which responds to national disasters. Over the years, he has participated as a volunteer on special NOVA crisis response teams sent to the sites of major disasters such as the Amtrack train wreck in Chase, Md. and the bus crash in Radcliff, Ky. He led trainings and debriefings with affected communities, and met with clergy to help them prepare for handling the numerous spiritual questions that would arise in the aftermath of the disasters.

Support for caregivers

Davis realizes that caregivers like himself also need support. His own support system is an informal network of pastor friends, hospital friends, and other people he can pick up the phone and call. In addition, he receives support from Farmington Baptist Church in Farmington, N.C., where he has been pastor for the last four years.

"I can leave the crisis mode and be with church family. I get nurturing and affection — it's a complete change for me. And it's a good reminder that what I am doing *is* a ministry."

For more information on the Forsyth County Sheriff's Department Victim Assistance Program, contact The Rev. Glenn G. Davis at:
3430 Stimpson Drive
Pfafftown, NC 27040
For information on the National Organization for Victim Assistance, contact NOVA at:
1757 Park Rd. N.W.
Washington, D.C. 20010

Appendix 4

Toolkits, Links and Resources

Concerns of Police Survivors (C.O.P.S.) makes the following material available to a department that has just suffered a loss:
https://www.concernsofpolicesurvivors.org/digital-materials
From their homepage at www.concernsofpolicesurvivors.org
On the survivor page there is a link to benefits by state.

Also under that digital-materials page is the first document compiled by C.O.P.S. in 1993…Susie Sawyer started the organization when a friend was killed in the line of duty.

More about C.O.P.S.' support for families can be found here:
https://irp-cdn.multiscreensite.com/ac5c0731/files/uploaded/support.pdf

National Fallen Firefighters Foundation (firehero.org)

National Law Enforcement Officers Memorial Fund (NLEOMF) https://nleomf.org/

Officer Down Memorial Page (ODMP) www.odmp.org

About the Authors

Rev. Glenn G. Davis, MDiv

Rev. Glenn Davis has served since 2016 as the Chaplain Director of the First Responder Chaplaincy Program (FRCP) in the FaithHealth Division of Atrium Health Wake Forest Baptist (AHWFB). The FRCP is a one-of-a-kind innovation as a hospital-based, community-focused model of chaplaincy delivering highly proactive, on-scene care to our most valuable and vulnerable public servants and their families.

Prior to moving to AHWFB and developing the FRCP, Chaplain Davis was the full-time Chaplain for the Forsyth County Sheriff's Office (FCSO) for over 27 years, serving as a member of the Command Staff while assisting the FCSO and other local and regional agencies and organizations. Currently, he and his team are proudly continuing to serve the FCSO as well as many other First Responders and stakeholders in Winston-Salem and Forsyth County. Expectations are that the FRCP will eventually grow to serve other communities within the Atrium Health network.

The FRCP provides on-call staff support and crisis intervention for law enforcement, other First Responder groups, and their family members as well as a broad range of survivors-victims-witnesses of crime and other catastrophic events. Chaplain Davis and his team routinely deploy 24/7/365 to assist law enforcement, fire, EMS and other organizations in the aftermath of critical incidents and to deliver traumatic messages while being alongside the First Responders who are also affected by these life-altering events. The team's embedded relationships with First Responder agencies offer many opportunities to teach wellness and resiliency throughout the community and build extensive webs of trust that are invaluable when communities are under stress and responding to multiple threats involving public safety.

Chaplain Davis continues to collaborate throughout the community assisting many groups with a particular focus on teaching First Responders but also clergy, congregational leaders and other care providers who seek to enhance their skill sets to better care for all our public servants and each other. Improving the crisis response readiness of faith communities, neighborhoods and workplaces is of vital importance given that all can be impacted by a broad range of traumatic events.

Chaplain Davis is an ordained Baptist minister and a graduate of the College of Charleston (BS) and Southeastern Baptist Theological Seminary (M.Div.) and the Clinical Pastoral Education (CPE) Residency Program at Atrium Health Wake Forest Baptist. Glenn is married to Patti Davis with whom he has a son, daughter, and granddaughter.

Teresa Cutts, PhD

Dr. Teresa Cutts completed her post-doctoral fellowship in Health Psychology from the University of Tennessee (UT) College of Medicine in 1987. From 1988 to 1994, she worked as a staff psychologist at Baptist Memorial Hospital. From 1993 to 2001, she was a private practitioner at Memphis Center for Women and Families, with a focus on health psychology. Since 1987, she served as a consultant to the NIH Gastroparesis multi-site consortium.

From 2001 to 2005, she was Director of Program Development at the Church Health Center, a comprehensive, faith-based health program for the under-served. She held a joint clinical appointment in Preventive Medicine and Psychiatry at UT, 2003–2008, University of Memphis' School of Public Health, 2009–2013, and still holds an appointment at Memphis Theological Seminary. She is a Visiting Professor at the University of Capetown's School of Family Medicine and Public Health and has co-authored/published numerous book chapters and articles.

In 2016, with colleagues from Stakeholder Health, she was co-editor and helped co-author many chapters in the book *Stakeholder Health: Insights from New Systems of Health*, as well as the 2019 *See2See Road Trip: Soundings* and *See2See Road Trip: Inland Sea* in 2020.

In 2005, she moved to Methodist Le Bonheur Healthcare's (MLH) Interfaith Health Program Center of Excellence in Faith and Health as Director of Research for Innovation. She worked explicitly in the area of evaluation and program development for Methodist's Memphis Model Congregational Health Network, Religious Health Assets mapping, and Integrated Health for congregations, community and clergy. She is the academic liaison to the Stakeholder Health learning collaborative. Dr. Cutts has served as PI or Co-PI on dozens of grants since 2001, including those funded by RWJF, CDC, Komen and Avon Foundations, working often on projects to improve health equity and the lives of the under-served and most vulnerable.

In 2013, Teresa was appointed as Research Assistant Professor, faculty at the Wake Forest School of Medicine's Public Health Sciences Division, where she serves as a researcher, program developer and more for the FaithHealth Division. She also holds appointments in the Maya Angelou Center for Health Equity. Since 2017, she has served as the PI for the Empowerment Project's homeless outreach and case management at WFSOM. She is married to Rev. Dr. Gary Gunderson and, between them, have four daughters and two grandsons.